I0135116

Alarmist Gatekeeping

Abortion

Dr Deborah Garratt PhD.

Printed in Australia

ISBN 978-0-9943524-1-5

For every woman silently grieving a loss and for my grandchildren, that a new and better culture awaits them in their adulthood.

Liam

Zoe

Joshua

Freya

Nate

"I have seen women make this decision dozens of times. I had even seen some of them suffer afterwards, but I always firmly believed it was because of their religious conflict or some radical pro-life guilt trip.

I never in a million years believed that their grief or sorrow was real, or that their beliefs that they felt pressured were genuine."

Penny, Social Worker

Dr Deborah Garratt

Foreword

When one ideological position dominates the discourse on any topic, covertly and overtly punishing the bearers of dissenting evidence and points of view, the price paid is loss of our individual freedom in the immediate, and the perversion of objective reality in the long-term. In the arena of abortion, the silencing and stifling of the advancement of science and the development of protocols to maximally benefit women are the sacrifices for forcing an ideologically-driven agenda for decades.

With the gift of this book, we can all breathe a long-overdue sigh of relief. Finally, a cohesive work that validates what so many of us have dealth with personally and professionally, explanations and labels for the players and components of a thoroughly entrenched phenomenon that has effectively robbed us of the ability to tackle the problem of abortion head on. This fascinating perspective merges the emic (insider) with the etic (outsider) perspectives with an expansive view facilitating a deep understanding of the powerful momentum with which this movement operates.

Dr Garratt's book also raises critical new questions that we should begin the process of addressing.

Firstly, what are the historical underpinnings that have allowed us to arrive where we are today?

Second, are there key players who have set alarmist gatekeeping into motion or has it emerged via a confluence of individuals and governing bodies who embrace common ideology?

Third, was this an organised, strategic plan of empowerment or did it evolve organically to take on the life it has now?

Fourth, what are the underlying motivations and are they even clearly discernible at this advanced stage?

Dr Garratt has provided the framework and understanding and now as a society of concerned individulas motivated to provide optimal care for women considering abortion, undergoing the procedure, and dealing with the personal and relational consequences, we have an ethical obligation to develop a strategy to implement change. The new paradigm must allow truth to emerge based on safe discourse wherein there is respect for all perspectives and freedom of expression. Moreover, a cultural shift is in order wherein this change is what the majority desire and work diligently to uphold.

We need courageous individuals to stand with Dr Garratt and insist the frightening evil of suppression that has resulted in proliferation of false information and irreparable harm to women, families, and society will no longer be tolerated.

Hope that the madness will one day end and future generations will benefit keeps many of us in the trenches calling for justice. With the release of this book, my prayer is that more and more people will have had enough and jump in with us. Of course, the pragmatic Dr Garratt is already thinking along these lines and is working on her next book, 'Gatebreaking: Countering Alarmist Gatekeeping', which she tantalises the reader with at the end of this book, noting it,

> *"...outlines concrete strategies to respond to and counter the disinformation and manipulation inherent in such controlled discourse. Above all, we must gain strength in numbers by refusing to self-censor and encouraging debate even when it makes us uncomfortable."*

Priscilla K. Coleman, PhD
Bowling Green State University
Bowling Green, Ohio, USA

Contents

Preface

This research did not set out as an examination of abortion discourse. The initial intent was to explore how practitioners interact with women who disclosed an abortion intent or experience. I expected to identify knowledge gaps or communication deficits that could inform the development of education packages so that practitioners were better resourced to support women.

Given that there is very little known about the interactions between practitioners and women on the issue of abortion, Grounded Theory was my chosen methodology; the ideal way to generate theory in unresearched fields. Grounded Theory dictates that the researcher must always follow the data rather than impose an agenda. In this case that data took me to very different places and to very different outcomes.

Initially recruiting practitioners from a wide range of those with whom women might come into contact—general practitioners, mental health nurses, social workers, psychologists, and counsellors—it quickly became apparent that knowledge about abortion was not high on the list of concerns of any of them.

By only the third interview, the data was pointing toward concerns about what it was appropriate to say, or what they felt 'allowed' to say, rather than whether they knew the information. Some practitioners were able to articulate very clearly what their concerns were. Others expressed a vague sense of uneasiness about what would be okay and who would know. Some were also able to identify at least some of the sources of such unease in the information they'd been relying on, yet others just expressed the need to censor information as "well you just know, don't you."

Some recognised that they intentionally self-censored: "*Oh, I would never say that because it's too risky*," and others could identify what they might not say, but accepted that it was just the norm: for example, "*well of course that would just be manipulative.*"

As the focus shifted from practitioner knowledge to broader concerns, I struggled with the enormity of the task ahead and also questioned whether I was going to be too close to the data, given my own involvement in the discourse. I had an article published in which I explored the challenges of being an "expert" in a field when undertaking Grounded Theory.[1] I also revealed my angst about engaging in the ideological aspect of abortion rather than simply being able to provide education.

> *It became clear that practitioners' interactions with clients were a direct result of the influences to which they were subject; and they were able to identify many of these influences from within the dominant discourse of abortion. I had spent a decade being critical of it [the dominant discourse] and its active silencing of the negative ways in which many women experienced abortion. While my own work was heavily censored and marginalised by advocates of the dominant discourse, I didn't yet understand either its power or consequences. I certainly lacked awareness of the pervasiveness of the*

---

1 Garratt, D. (2018). Reflections on being an expert. *Grounded Theory Review*, 1(17). http://groundedtheoryreview.com/2018/12/27/reflections-on-being-an-expert/

dominant messaging or how powerful it was in its ability to censor and to silence. I had lamented my own inability to gain traction in mainstream media and had dealt with significant hostility and censoring from ideological advocates unhappy with my approach. However, I had attributed the inability of my work to gain mainstream attention to my lack of marketing skills and contacts.

As the theory developed, the professional challenges I faced at this time were significant, as my awareness of all the ways in which I had tackled issues of education, of supporting women, and of managing the dominant discourse seemed ineffective. My desire to educate practitioners into being more knowledgeable and therefore supportive of women was founded on false assumptions that education was all that was necessary. The discourse was more powerful and more pervasive than I had imagined. It was also more dangerous to my research than I had anticipated.

Encouraged by my supervisor and my Grounded Theory mentor, I ventured on and the theory of Alarmist Gatekeeping emerged. This book is primarily the product of that PhD research, including the analysis of thousands of data from many sources such as interviews, mainstream and social media, political documents, professional body statements and more. I have included a Glossary at the end of the book to explain terms that are unique to this theory and to the topic of abortion.

The book is greatly enhanced by the stories shared with me by women I have met over the past twenty years. My hope is that these women will have a sense that I have represented their experiences with enough depth and compassion and that the sharing of their stories will help them to create a different meaning in their own lives. It is only because of the privilege of walking alongside so many of them that this book can exist.

A Pervasive Power

How they control what you think, say, and do.

Alarmist Gatekeeping is a theory that explains the phenomenon of Dominant Discoursing on abortion in Australia. It identifies the people who participate in it, and reveals the very real and disturbing consequences for women. As a process, Alarmist Gatekeeping is inherently manipulative in its effect, given its power to control the actions of people, the 'acceptable' language, and even legislative change based on Disinformation. It stops doctors from effectively screening women for risk factors or from offering alternative options. It prevents women from receiving information about the harms of abortion. It results in people losing careers and having their reputations tarnished or ruined if they speak against abortion.

Alarmist Gatekeeping comprises two distinct strategies—Alarmist Recruitment and Perspective Gatekeeping—which work together to reinforce each other and perpetuate a cycle of disinformation and censorship. On one side, Alarmist Recruitment recruits you to a general cause of women's rights while convincing you that without your support desperate women will die. On the other side, Perspective Gatekeeping restricts your access to alternative facts, ensures you don't question that which is presented as 'truth' and makes very public the consequences for those who do.

In order to understand the serious consequences of Alarmist Gatekeeping and the complex ways in which the process works, this first chapter gives an overview of the interacting elements and the people involved in perpetuation of the Dominant Discourse.

Power of Pervasiveness

The Dominant Discourse on abortion in Australia, as in many western countries, very strongly advocates for abortion. The message that women must have access to abortion as a human right is pervasive across education, professional bodies, media, and politics. It has become so ingrained that few question it and if they do, it is generally at significant personal or professional cost.

When a Dominant Message is perpetuated across the range of influences to which one is subject, the power of its effect multiplies. The more often a message is heard by a person, the more likely it is to be believed and adopted.[2] The psychological process of believing that which is already believed or which is heard more often, as opposed to new or contradictory information, also assists in perpetuating the Dominant Messaging.[3]

A phenomenon called the Illusory-Truth Effect[4] demonstrates that repetition creates familiarity along with a tendency to believe something as true based on familiarity rather than veracity. This means that the more often we hear something, the more likely we are to believe it to be true even if we never verify it.

---

2 Moons, W., Mackie, D. and Garcie-Marques, T. (2007). The Impact of Repetition-Induced Familiarity on Agreement with Weak and Strong Arguments. *Journal of Personality and Social Psychology*, 96(1):32-44.

3 Begg, I., Anas, A., and Farinacci, S. (1992). Dissociation of Processes in Belief: Source Recollection, Statement Familiarity, and the Illusion of Truth. *Journal of Experimental Psychology*, 121(2):446-458.

4 Hasher, L., Goldstein, D., and Toppino, T. (1977). Frequency and the Conference of Referential Validity. *Journal of Verbal Learning and Verbal Behavior*, 16:107-112.

Some practitioners in this study would state that they 'knew' something without really knowing how or why they knew it to be true:

> *"Well you just know don't you... that you can't talk about it [abortion harm]. It's like an unwritten rule; we all know." (Mental Health Nurse)*

In this way, the messaging of the Dominant Discourse has been internalised in no small degree, and for the most part goes unquestioned. The personal and professional risks of questioning can run high in the presence of any perceived threat to abortion rights.

Recruitment to a common cause is relatively easy in a setting of pervasive messaging. Recruitment entails ensuring an agreeable general cause, often accompanied by Alarmist statements which are either greatly exaggerated or even fabricated. The process of abstraction of actual experience to a generalised statement has been called "strategic ambiguity" and this promotes what Eisenberg[5] terms a "unified diversity."

In effect this means it is easy to get people to agree on a vague, abstract message with some consensus. In Alarmist Gatekeeping on abortion we see statements such as *"women have the right to control their own bodies"* or *"women have the right to equality."* Both statements are abstract and vague, implying a cause with which people of good will can agree.

Such statements may often be in the company of Alarmist Disinformation such as:

> *"Millions of women die each year from a lack of access to abortion."*

---

5 Eisenberg, E. (1984). Ambiguity as Strategy in Organisational Communication. *Communication Monographs*, 51:227-242.

… from Australian abortion advocate Leslie Cannold (the Disinformation in this statement is addressed later).

Few people are prepared to say "no" to the Recruitment statements and many simply believe the Alarmist Disinformation, particularly when it is repeated so often across many different platforms. In the case of abortion, the same or similar messaging is pervasive. It is repeated by media, professional bodies, educational institutions, political discussion and many more.

Disinformation is very common in the Dominant Messaging and it is almost impossible for the general public to discern the facts when Experts perpetuate it. So who are the players and who determines the Experts?

The Players

The general view is that there are two polarised opinions on abortion, pro-life and pro-choice, with each side having its labels for themselves and the 'other.' Pro-choice people often describe pro-life as anti-choice and pro-life people may describe pro-choice as pro-abortion.

What is revealed in Alarmist Gatekeeping is that there are far more complex and nuanced positions on the issue and the Dominant Group doesn't necessarily hold the most popular view. The Dominant Group does, however, hold the power to label others according to whether they find the person or their messages in keeping with the desired perspective.

Identifying these players is an important finding as it gives some insight into both the strengths and challenges inherent in effective discussion around abortion. Understanding the way in which each type responds to the Discourse may help in developing strategies for the way we present information and for addressing the issues of self-censorship that often leave women lacking information and support.

The three types of people, Adherents, Incognisants, and

Dissidents, are broad representations of the population in terms of their awareness, compliance, and agreement or disagreement with the Dominant Messaging.

Adherents are the dominant voices of the Discourse. They hold the power to decide who the Experts are, what constitutes 'acceptable' information, and whether another person or organisation belongs to their ranks.

Adherents idealise the concept of abortion rights, appearing to hold this principle in higher regard than whether individual women enact abortion as a right or whether they instead feel pressured, coerced, or have negative experiences. The principle of abortion rights is usually promoted as being one of the last vestiges of inequality and lack of freedom[6] or as "intimately tied to gender equality."[7]

Stories which may paint abortion in a negative light, whether presented by women themselves of their own experiences, or by professionals simply presenting evidence of adverse effects, will be met with swift denials. Such denials are accompanied by processes of Discrediting the messenger in order to further undermine the message, an element of Perspective Gatekeeping.

There are two types of Adherents; those who know they are dispensing Disinformation (false information) and those who disseminate the information believing it to be true. The former deliberately falsify information because they consider that some facts may threaten abortion rights. We assume that certain Adherents such as abortion providers are in this category. The latter type fall into the category of people who have been manipulated and now believe that what they say is the truth. In some ways their words may hold greater power than those who intentionally

6 Sifris, R. and Belton, S. (2017). Abortion and Human Rights. *Health and Human Rights Journal,* 19(1):209-220.
7 Plibersek, T. (2019). Foreword. In Swinn, L. (ed.) *Choice Words: A Collection of Stories About Abortion,* Allen and Unwin.

deceive. Rigotti[8] identifies greater manipulative impact when *"an already manipulated person aims at convincing another."* He goes on to say that manipulation from this group could be at least in part unintentional, given that they themselves have been manipulated. It makes sense that we may be less convinced by someone deliberately lying as we sense some subtle cues that are not present when someone believes they are telling the truth, thereby making the latter more convincing.

Not only do Adherents represent themselves as the ultimate authority on abortion, they also give themselves the only authority to decide who can be considered an Expert (Adherent-labelled Experts will be recognised throughout by capitalisation).

Van Dijk[9] says people with the power to exercise social control of others *"need to satisfy personal and social criteria that enable them to influence others."* Expert status is determined primarily by the person's strict adherence to upholding abortion rights and by their ability to hold some influence whether in the media or by virtue of their professional position or qualification.

They may be abortion providers or those in positions of influence on behalf of abortion advocating organisations, or mainstream media or social media engagement. You will see stories throughout this book demonstrating that status as an Expert is very tenuous and Adherents have no tolerance for anything other than total commitment to the principle. The major criteria for being an Expert is one's ability to always toe the line and never say anything that may threaten the principle of abortion rights, even inadvertently.

We might expect that such professionals have a duty to be

---

8 Rigotti, E. (2005). Towards a Typology of Manipulative Processes. In: L. de Saussure and P. Schultz, ed., *Manipulation and Ideologies in the Twentieth Century: Discourse, Language, Mind.* John Benjamins Publishing.
9 Van Dijk, T. (2006). Discourse and Manipulation. *Discourse and Society,* Vol 17(2): 359-383.

well-informed about the breadth of experience and research in which they are purported to be Expert. However, this is not always the case. It is not the aim of this thesis to imbue Influential People designated as Experts with malicious intent in their contribution to the discourse, but rather to explain how their role adds to the power of manipulative consequence. De Saussure[10] tells us that even a *"weakly entertained belief stated with great authority can be manipulative."* In the setting of a Dominant Discourse, such as that of abortion rights, the strength of belief appears to be the belief in the Principle, the upholding of rights, more so than the veracity of the spoken facts. The 'Great Authority' within abortion discoursing rests with Adherents, promoted as the Experts and trusted by the public to provide necessary and truthful information.

Adherents don't perceive any professional or personal risk in upholding abortion advocacy. However, even one small slip can mean they topple from Adherent to Dissident and experience the painful processes of being Discredited and Out-Grouped.

Dissidents do not necessarily hold a view against abortion in principle and may even self-identify as pro-choice.

When Australian journalist Rita Panahi tweeted her opinion on abortion at full term gestation, saying, *"I'm pro-choice but there's no justification for abortion at eight months when the child could be born alive,"* she was quickly advised, *"then you're not pro-choice"* by an Adherent Expert.

Nobody is granted the privilege of self-identifying in an environment where every piece of information is filtered through its threat to abortion rights. There is zero tolerance among Adherents

---

10 de Saussure, L. (2005). Manipulation and Cognitive Pragmatics: Preliminary Hypotheses. In de Saussure Louis and Peter Schulz (Eds), *Manipulation and Ideologies in the Twentieth Century: Discourse, Language, Mind.* Amsterdam-Philadelphia, John Benjamins, 113-146.

for allowing such dissent among their ranks.

There are also Dissidents who hold views against abortion and who actively work to bring about change, and there are those who choose not to engage at all due to perceived risks. This type generally has a high awareness of the risks they may face in speaking out, and of the challenges in overcoming the censorship of information in the mainstream.

Incognisants are the most populous group sitting in the middle ground. They are likely to have shown little interest in discussing or questioning the subject of abortion even if personally affected. They are most likely to have simply internalised the messaging of the Dominant Discoursing as true; that abortion rights must be upheld, otherwise women suffer. If an Incognisant has an abortion and does experience suffering, they are more likely to accept that their suffering is not connected to abortion and for this reason may not even talk about it. They will accept the Discrediting of Dissidents due to the harm Adherents tell them is caused to women. They may choose not to believe Dissident information in favour of listening to the Experts.

If Incognisants are exposed to information that makes them uncomfortable, they will generally fall back into the comfort of believing Adherents' denials rather than explore the discomfort and seek their own facts. Because Incognisants internalise the Dominant Discourse as true, even if they have concerns or doubts, they are more likely to respond positively to questioning about abortion availability and rights. The social and psychological processes that contribute to this will be unpacked through the stories that follow.

*"I knew deep in my heart that abortion was not
something I wanted to do. I went to my appointment, my boyfriend came with me. I was pretty sure
that at the last minute I would panic and decide to
keep my baby. But I was sedated and given pretty
powerful pain medication that prevented me from
thinking rationally. I don't remember too much
about the procedure. It started before I even realized it. I was supposed to say something at the very
last possible moment. That way my boyfriend could
at least see I tried. But those powerful meds made
me lose the ability to do this.*

*By the time I'd realized what had happened it was
too late to take it back. I didn't feel the real effects
until the next day once the drugs had completely
worn off. I was devastated. I still am. I am broken.
I don't know how to cope. Part of me wants to die.
Living without my lovely baby seems like a terrible
existence. I don't know where to go from here. I do
know that I will never be the same again" (Nala)*

Alarmist Recruitment:

The Pervasive Power of Alarm and Deceit

"If we are able to influence people's minds—for example, their knowledge, attitudes or ideologies— we indirectly may control some of their actions, as we know from persuasion and manipulation."[11]

Discussions around abortion access and availability are framed by Alarmist Gatekeeping in profoundly negative and alarmist terms as though every situation where a woman may consider abortion is potentially life-limiting or hazardous. The fact that most abortions in Australia are undertaken for psychosocial concerns is minimised, ignored or denied, while the emphasis is given to the most extreme and most rare circumstances. The term psychosocial encompasses a wide variety of reasons including not having enough resources (financial or other resources), feeling concerned about keeping a job or continuing education, and feeling unsupported or too young or too old. It does not include

---

11 van Dijk, T. (2015). Critical Discourse Analysis. In Tannen, D., Hamilton, H. and Schiffrin, D. *The Handbook of Discourse Analysis* (2nd ed., 466-485). John Wiley and Sons Inc.

concerns around physical or serious mental health of the woman or of the unborn baby.[12]

Abortion is also often promoted as the answer to saving the lives of women who may die during pregnancy or during or shortly after birth. This is a typical headline in an online news article lamenting the lack of abortion:

> *Pregnancy can kill. No one should be forced to give birth against their will.*[13]

The by-line makes the intention of alarm even clearer:

> *Everyone should be able to decide whether to risk maternal mortality.*

The article contains stories of women who died from pregnancy-related complications including infections following childbirth and a cardiac condition which worsened during pregnancy. While aborting any one of these pregnancies may have meant the woman didn't die, there is no indication that abortion was requested, considered, or wanted by any of these women. Likewise, Adherent Expert Leslie Cannold stated on SBS television that

> *"..millions of women die each year from a lack of access to abortion."*[14]

She went on to talk about the millions who die in childbirth in developing countries. Not only is this figure Alarmist, and an example of Disinformation, it also conflates two unrelated issues given that the majority of women dying in these countries do so

---

12 I use the term "unborn baby" throughout given that this is the most common term women would use when talking about their pregnancy.

13 Valenti, J. (9 Aug 2017). Pregnancy Can Kill. No One Should be Forced to Give Birth Against Their Will. *The Guardian*. https://www.theguardian.com/commentisfree/2017/aug/09/pregnancy-can-kill-right-to-chose-jessica-valenti

14 *The Feed*, SBS Television.

from a lack of knowledge and resources to manage infection and haemorrhage, not a lack of abortion.[15] In 2015, maternal deaths during and following pregnancy and childbirth numbered around 303,000 worldwide, most of which were from the preventable causes cited above. There is no suggestion that the women dying in these circumstances are doing so because they could not access abortion or ever considered abortion as an option.

Another oft-repeated statement that is both misleading and alarmist is how much safer abortion is than childbirth.

> *"She told me it would be safer than having a baby. I'm pretty sure she told me that having the abortion would be ten times safer than staying pregnant or giving birth or something like that. What she didn't say, and what I didn't think of in my panic to just get it all over with is that if I stayed pregnant, I would actually have a baby and that maybe that risk would be worth it." (Lena)*

When stated by Experts, it has added power regardless of the fact that there is credible evidence to support the opposite assertion; childbirth is safer than abortion.[16] One Expert, an obstetrician/gynaecologist in a regional area of Australia, has stated several times publicly in the media that "abortion is 100 times safer than childbirth." While actively Disinforming in this way, he concurrently accuses Dissidents of being misleading and alarmist when they express concerns about the potential adverse effects of abortion.

> *"Anti-abortion groups will often claim women*

---

15 World Health Organization (19 Sept 2018). Maternal Mortality: Key Facts. *World Health Organization.* https://www.who.int/news-room/fact-sheets/detail/maternal-mortality
16 Gissler, M., Berg, C., Bouvier-Colle, M. H. and Buekens, P. (2005). Injury Deaths, Suicides and Homicides Associated with Pregnancy, Finland 1987–2000, *European Journal of Public Health*, 15(5):459–463.

aren't warned of the risks but neglect to state that abortion at any gestation is safer than childbirth."[17]

"Abortion is much safer than a vaginal delivery, and infinitely safer than a caesarean. We still see women who die in childbirth in Australia. People haven't got that possibility even in their mind."[18]

It is worth considering whether the impact of Disinformation about the relative safety of abortion versus childbirth provides reassurance to women who have already decided on abortion or whether it further alarms those who are undecided.

"I was already pretty scared about having a baby. My friend's mum died after she had my friend's sister. My friend and I were six at the time and I always imagined it as a horrifying blood bath with lots of screaming even though I have no idea what really happened. When he told me this [the abortion] would be safer than having a baby, all I had in my head was the screaming I'd imagined." (Naomi)

The issue of late-term abortion is one of more considerable discomfort for many people. Community attitude surveys demonstrate less support for abortion at later gestations especially for reasons of social or economic concern.

In the State of Victoria, where abortion is available throughout the entirety of pregnancy, around half of all post-twenty-week terminations are undertaken for psychosocial reasons. In 2017, the last year for which statistics are available at the time of

---

17 Rushton, G. (15 Mar 2017). We spent the day at a pro-life service for women with 'problem pregnancies.' *BuzzFeed News*. https://www.buzzfeed.com/ginarushton/priceless-house

18 Paxman, A. (20 Jul 2017). Later-term abortions: Stigma versus reality. *Sydney Morning Herald*. https://www.smh.com.au/lifestyle/laterterm-abortions-stigma-versus-reality-20170720-gxf4ym.html

writing, there were a total of 323 post-20 week abortions, with 140 being for psychosocial indications. Of this total, 28 resulted in neonatal deaths, meaning that the babies were born alive and then died.[19] In the decade between 2008 and 2017 there were 1595 post-20-week terminations for psychosocial reasons in Victoria alone, along with 364 babies born alive following late termination. These are not facts that Adherents like to have in the public sphere. The discomfort generated by the idea of a healthy baby being terminated is addressed in a later chapter.

Disinformation is a common and important practice of Adherents, given the public discomfort with truth about abortion. The public is more inclined to support late-term abortion in cases of severe foetal abnormality, or where the mother's life may be at risk. This means they are more likely to respond affirmatively to questions about abortion access during pregnancy, based on their beliefs that late-term abortions only occur in these extreme circumstances. It is the norm that information to the contrary, even when evidence is provided, will be subject to vehement objection in social media discussions.

When we read information about abortion, we reasonably expect the Experts to have accurate knowledge on the issue and will be inclined to believe them. They would be considered Experts by the general public, the media, and politicians. In spite of the publicly available information, Disinformation delivered by abortion providers and presented in print media and submissions to government are everywhere:

> *"Viable babies are not aborted. When terminations at or after 20 weeks' gestation do occur, they are rare and tragic cases—such as an extreme*

19 Table detailing data by year since 1999 available at: https://www.realchoices.org.au/research/abortion/late-term-abortion-statistics/vic/

> *maternal condition or late diagnosis of a lethal foe-*
> *tal abnormality."[20]*

> *"26 weeks gestation is "far above the upper world-*
> *wide limit of abortion."[21]*

The above statements were found in official submissions to government enquiries by people who are considered Expert in the
area and which significantly influenced legislative change. The
result of legislation based on such Expert Disinformation further
perpetuates the Dominant Messaging. People believe if it's in the
law it must be true and correct.

Swiss language educator Louis de Saussure suggests that not
only do speakers sometimes deliver Disinformation in order to
manipulate, but sometimes also withhold certain relevant information, or fabricate relevance of information that may not actually be relevant in a particular context.[22] When defining a deliberately misleading communication, Swedish philosopher and
epistemologist Andreas Stokke[23] says:

> *"I propose that to mislead is to disrupt the pursuit*
> *of the goal of inquiry, that is, to prevent the progress*
> *of inquiry from approaching the discovery of how*
> *things are, i.e. 'the pursuit of truth."*

Stokke's proposal suggests one of intention in disruption, an intent
to prevent reality or truth from being known which involves not
just intentional lying, but misleading, evading, or withholding of

20 Submission No. 753 to Senate Enquiry into Decriminalisation of Abortion in
Queensland, 2016, submitted by anonymous self-described "GP and Specialist Sexual
Health Physician"
21 Grimes, D. R. (3 Apr 2018). Myths and lies about abortion must
be debunked. *The Irish Times*. https://www.irishtimes.com/opinion/
myths-and-lies-about-abortion-must-be-debunked-1.3448176
22 de Saussure, Manipulation and Cognitive Pragmatics.
23 Stokke, Andrea. (2016). Lying and Misleading in Discourse. *Philosophical Review*,
125(1):83-134.

information. Huckin[24] agrees that in the framing of public issues, what isn't said may be as important as what is said. In the framing of a topic, a speaker will mention some relevant issues while ignoring others so as to provide a particular perspective.

He provides three criteria for determining whether the omission of some detail can be considered manipulative: deception, intentionality, and advantage. He claims that it is deceptive to leave out or conceal information that could be considered relevant to understanding, in order to give prominence to other information, which then does not provide a balanced view. We see this occurring in examples where Experts deliver Disinformation or distract from a particular question by answering something else.

Let's look at some of the ways in which Experts use deception and omission to avoid truth-telling when asked directly about late-term abortion. In a BuzzFeed[25] article professing to expose the lies and myths of anti-choice rhetoric, Experts are asked a number of questions including,

> *Does decriminalising abortion allow babies to be killed up until the moment of birth?*

The responses from Experts to this question include:

> *"This is an anti-choice talking point and is untrue and completely unsupported by evidence. Most abortions take place before 12 weeks' gestation."*

This response contains a combination of Perspective Gatekeeping manifested by OutGrouping and Discrediting (it is "an anti-choice talking point"), and Alarmist Recruitment by

---

24 Huckin, T. (2002). Textual silence and the discourse of homelessness. *Discourse and Society,* 13(3):347-372.

25 Rushton, G. (30 Jan 2018). This is what reproductive health experts think about the comments section on abortion stories. *BuzzFeed.* https://www.buzzfeed.com/ginarushton/experts-read-the-comments

Disinformation (it is "untrue"), and obfuscation (changing the subject to early abortions).

> *"Later-term abortions are very rare, with the consensus figure being that about 1% of abortions fall into this category. Later-term abortions take place in a hospital setting in complex, challenging and extreme circumstances."*

Abstraction is used effectively here to draw attention from the question through what some researchers have defined as the "intentional use of imprecise language,"[26] also called equivocation. While the response does not directly address the question under discussion, this fact may bypass the processing of many who hear it so they don't notice the original question wasn't answered.

> *"This is a myth. There are areas in the world where, in theory, abortion until birth could be allowed... there are almost always strong caveats about the situation needing to be one of life or death for either the mother or foetus."*

This response from the BuzzFeed article is another equivocating abstraction designed to be misleading, combined with Disinformation ("*this is a myth*"). The Expert does not directly say that this can't or doesn't happen, conceding that it might happen somewhere in the world, however leaving the impression that this doesn't include Australia, the country in question. He also uses the words "*almost always*" which allows some backtracking if he was to be confronted with this as Disinformation.

We can see from the above examples the way in which both direct and indirect deception and abstraction is used to draw our attention

---

26 Hamilton, M. A. and Mineo, P.J. (1998). A Framework for Understanding Equivocation. *Journal of Language and Social Psychology*, 17(1):3-35.

to other aspects that are indirectly related to the original question. It is a kind of 'political speak' that many don't see through, but it can leave you feeling a little uncomfortable or dissatisfied.

A Dangerous Language

*"My friend is having a baby... a baby. How come
she is having a baby, and I just stopped a pregnancy
which apparently had nothing to do with a baby?"
(Mel)*

Language is a powerful tool that can be used to distort, manipulate, minimise, and alarm. It can also be used to dehumanise and disconnect as is the case when the way in which an unborn baby is labelled is dependent on a person's perceived feelings about it.

Controlling language is a strategic aspect of Alarmist Gatekeeping designed to confuse thinking, override one's defences, depersonalise, and dehumanise. Every thinking person knows and every human biology textbook confirms that what grows inside the womb of a pregnant woman is a human being. Control of language in this way seeks to create more disconnect for a woman between herself and her baby. This comes at a time when such connection may be exactly what she needs in order to gather the resources and strengths to face what for many women is an extreme pressure toward abortion.

In November 2011 a Melbourne couple made what was considered a difficult decision to end the life of one of their unborn twins at 32 weeks of pregnancy due to a congenital abnormality. On the day of the procedure, ultrasounds were performed to ensure that the life of the healthy twin was preserved while the unhealthy twin's heart was stopped. For some reason, the healthy twin's heart was stopped with a cardiac injection meant for the other twin. Both babies were subsequently delivered by caesarean section with the remaining live (but unhealthy) twin being terminated at the same time (although details are sketchy about the method undertaken for this).

This was a tragedy. This couple, excitedly expecting two babies then making a heartbreaking decision to end the life of one, went home without any babies at all. The media headlines screamed outrage, as did many members of the public:

> *Medical bungle at Royal Women's Hospital kills healthy fetus.*[27]

> *Oz hospital 'accidently' terminates healthy fetus.*[28]

> *Tragic mix-up in which a baby was mistakenly aborted in Melbourne will be investigated.*[29]

The first article entitled "Medical Bungle" has a fine print statement at the bottom which reads:

> *Originally published as "Parents'pain after bungle kills healthy baby."*

It is as though people were confused about whether this was actually the life of a baby and if so, what do we do about the language

---

27 Drill, S. (24 Nov 2011). Medical Bungle at Royal Women's Hospital Kills Healthy Fetus. *News.com.au.*

28 NDTV (24 Nov 2011). Oz Hospital 'Accidentally' Terminates Healthy Foetus. *NDTV.* https://www.ndtv.com/world-news/oz-hospital-accidently-terminates-healthy-foetus-566473

29 Akerman, P. and Ferguson, J. (24 Nov 2011). Tragic Mix-Up in Which a Baby was Mistakenly Aborted in Melbourne will be Investigated. *The Australian.*

so as not to risk abortion rights?

One of the interesting aspects of reporting of the incident was the outcry from the public in social media commentary. People were rightly horrified that this healthy baby could be "accidentally" killed. Here was a missed opportunity to have talked about all of the healthy babies "killed" in terminations every year and to have raised awareness of the ways in which such "killing" is provided as a solution to the social problems of women.

In the same state of Victoria that year, the lives of 183 healthy babies were terminated after 20 weeks, 11 of them after 28 weeks, a gestation at which survival was the most likely outcome.[30] There were no news headlines, no outrage, no public outcry for these babies or their parents. There was nothing but utter complete silence in the name of "rights" and "choice." In fact, every year in Victoria there are around the same number of physically healthy mothers losing physically healthy babies to abortion. People are often shocked when they hear this yet, as we have seen, the strategies within Alarmist Gatekeeping will allow most of those people to comfortably ignore and dismiss the information as nothing more than a fabrication, even when provided with the statistical evidence.

Adherents will often insist that a "baby" doesn't exist until after birth yet will also interchangeably use the terms "foetus" and "baby" in their own discourse. One obstetrician and maternal-foetal medicine specialist, in her submission to Queensland parliament on the decriminalisation of abortion, explains the process of late-term abortion:

"The patient is contacted, and an induced foetal demise procedure is performed so that the baby is

30 Consultative Council on Obstetric and Paediatric Mortality and Morbidity (CCOPMM) (2014). *2010 and 2011 Victoria's Mothers and Babies: Victoria's Maternal, Perinatal, Child and Adolescent Mortality.* State of Victoria, Melbourne.

not born alive following the procedure. "[31]

She goes on to talk about the importance of counselling, educa-tion, and support for women considering late-term abortion. Yet she also criticises the potential waiting time for an ethics com-mittee to approve an abortion, saying the patient invariably wants the whole procedure over as quickly as possible. As though this doctor doesn't see her own words, she also suggests that "care-ful consideration should be given to terminology used in any legislation."

Adherents used the same confused terminology even when arguing against the proposed legislation, Zoe's Law, a law to allow a person to be prosecuted if an unborn baby is killed in the course of a crime. Zoe[32] was the name given to the unborn baby of a woman who was hit by a vehicle when she was 32 weeks pregnant. Zoe was subsequently delivered stillborn by caesar-ean section. At the time of the debate about this proposed law, Adherent organisations sent letters, spoke at events, and released statements primarily focused on what they perceived to be the risk to abortion rights if such a law were to pass. They also found it challenging to stick to their own permitted language:[33]

> *"..tragically lost her daughter in a motor vehicle accident."*

> *"..the circumstances under which (these parents) lost their babies are tragic."*

---

31 Sekar, R. (2016). Submission to Senate Enquiry Decriminalisation of Abortion, Queensland.
32 Barrowclough, N. (9 May 2017). Zoe's Law: Meet the NSW Mother Fighting to Rec-ognise Death of Foetuses over 20 Weeks Old as a Crime. *Marie Claire*. https://www.marie-claire.com.au/zoes-law-nsw-mother-fighting-to-recognise-death-of-foetuses-as-crime
33 Fernandez, M. (30 Oct 2014). *Women's Electoral Lobby*. Letter to NSW parliamentar-ian expressing "deep concern" about Zoe's Law.

"..the loss of a foetus can be a tragedy causing great grief and loss."

"..the redefinition of a foetus as a living person infringes on the rights of women seeking abortion."

Even though the wording of the proposed Bill allowed exceptions for abortion, Adherents remained adamant that the threat to abortion was too great:

"This bill is unnecessary and presents a real risk to women's reproductive rights by giving legal personhood to a foetus."[34]

Leslie Cannold, Adherent Expert, lamented that even referring to the law by a name made it too personal, as though the loss of any woman's baby is ever not a personal issue. Of course, what she means is that it sounds too human and imbuing a foetus with humanness is a threat to abortion.

"Foetal personhood laws set the foetus in opposition to the woman in whose body it is residing. Stop calling it "Zoe's" law. It makes it too personal."[35]

The concept of the rights of an unborn baby and the rights of a woman being in opposition is often foundational to Adherents' arguments as though only one can ever "win." It completely disavows any relationship or connection between the woman and her child. Most women see the unborn baby they are carrying as not only human, but many seek to know the sex so that they can give the baby a name, and talk to and about the baby from a relational perspective.

---

34 McGowan, M. (17 Nov 2018). Revived "Zoe's law" bill a risk to women's abortion rights, warn pro-choice groups. *The Guardian*. https://www.theguardian.com/australia-news/2018/nov/17/revived-zoes-law-bill-a-risk-to-womens-abortion-rights-warn-pro-choice-groups
35 Cannold, L. (23 Sept 2015). Talk given at SS&A Club Albury.

Inconsistencies and euphemisms create a confusion in our minds that can make us uncomfortable. When uncomfortable, we tend to look for the familiar to fall back on. Experts provide us that cushion with reassurances that of course women need abortion and of course those terrible stories told by those terrible people don't actually exist.

There are other more subtle ways in which language has been used over the years to both describe abortion and to recruit people to the cause. Consider the words "termination of pregnancy," for example. From a practical point of view a pregnancy terminates with miscarriage, abortion, and birth. It is a relatively benign term that suggests the ending of a process of pregnancy, which it does. However it leaves out some important information about what that entails. References to abortion procedures often use "pregnancy" as a noun to describe what is removed from a woman during termination. For example:

> *"A doctor uses gentle suction to remove the pregnancy from the uterus."[36]*

This language, as well as language describing medical abortion as a miscarriage, is designed to lessen the emotional impact and distract from the reality. The problem is that an abortion is an emotional act that many women understand at some point as having severed an important relationship, one that perhaps wasn't considered at the time.

Slogans, too, have been an integral aspect of abortion advocacy since the early days of activism. Many people hear the slogans and accept the broader meaning and messaging that has been ascribed to them by Adherents. For example:

> *Every child a wanted child.*

---

36 Explanation of surgical abortion by Marie Stopes on their website: https://www.marie-stopes.org.au/abortion/surgical-abortion/

This reinforces the notion that women seeking abortions don't want their babies, as opposed to seeing abortion as a solution to the problem of their circumstances. Along with the concept of a "wanted child" comes the Disinformation that "unwanted" children are somehow less worthy and at greater risk of abuse or neglect. Yet there is no evidence to support the idea that abused children are generally considered for abortion during pregnancy or that women denied abortion go on to abuse children. The "wantedness" concept also commodifies children in a way that sees them as property rather than as a person in relationship to another person (their mother, father, extended family) and as a human being.

Of course, there is also the commonly used slogan "the right to choose" which denotes that women are freely and autonomously making a choice from valid options. Or the "control of one's own body" when in fact once a pregnancy has begun there are two bodies involved. This is particularly pertinent when such control of one's own body is only seen as relevant when such control means bringing an end to pregnancy through abortion rather than continuing a pregnancy.

A study of Australian obstetricians explored the ethical issues created by the use of technologies such as ultrasound.[37] On the one hand we have doctors acknowledging that women will do everything in their power to save their unborn babies:

> *"The obstetricians commented that almost with no exceptions, women would go through a great deal and put up with inconvenience, discomfort, pain and even risks to their own health in order to protect the health of their fetus."*

37 Edvardsson, K., Small, R., Lalos, An., Persson, M., and Mogren, I. (2015). Ultrasound's "Window on the Womb" Brings Ethical Challenges for Balancing Maternal and Fetal Health Interests: Obstetrician's Experiences in Australia. *BMC Medical Ethics*, 16:31.

On the other hand, doctors may need to "contain" women's desires to save their babies which could be considered a way of denying them their "choice" and bodily autonomy:

> *Some of the time they just say: do whatever you can for the baby, and they really don't listen to you saying there are these downsides.*
>
> *There is that maternal selflessness so we may need to contain it, you know, in some ways saying no, this is too much, you know?"*

It is clear that both bodily autonomy and control of one's body are integral to arguments to promote abortion and for that we even manipulate language, yet the right to such control is rescinded when a woman doesn't want to end her pregnancy.

We can see that the control and manipulation of language has specific intent to draw attention from the reality of abortion and the reality of why women consider abortion. Language is used to disconnect women from what is going on inside their bodies, to ignore relationship, as though the entity within is an uninvited stranger, rather than a human being created within them.

For too many women, this language eases their angst at a time when they feel desperate and allows them to do something they might ordinarily not consider. For too many women, once the abortion is done, their hormones settle, the relief that is often experienced early on has passed, and reality sets in. It is this time when they are more confronted by what really happened, what they have done, and how they succumbed to the "choice."

"One of my friends posted something on her facebook about Zoe's law in New South Wales. She read about how it would stop women being able to have abortions and she kept saying how terrible that was. I read the story of how Zoe's law came about and I felt so sad for that mother (that her baby was killed by a drunk driver). She wanted her baby and someone killed it and she can't get any justice and now people are trying to say that her baby can't be valued because someone else might not want theirs?

My friend doesn't know what I did to my baby. She doesn't even know I was ever pregnant and I don't know if I could tell her without also telling her the horrible, horrible truth that I wish women couldn't have abortions. I wish no woman could ever do it, because if they couldn't then my baby would be here. I wish people would understand that just because the Zoe's Law mum wanted her baby doesn't mean some of us didn't too.

And that if it wasn't so damn bloody easy to get one and people didn't fill your head with so many lies about how bad it would be to be a mother then I would have been one by now. It's like it's all about rights to have an abortion, but what about my rights to know how this would feel? What about my rights to not feel pushed into it? When I rang the abortion clinic, and then rang someone they referred me to talk about how bad I felt they just kept reminding me it was my decision. I know it was. But I also know it wasn't.

If I didn't know enough about what might happen... If all those people had shut up and given me a chance to think, then it wouldn't have been my decision... never!!

All this crap about choice is bullshit. I'm sorry but it is. It's even worse than that but I don't think you'll print it.

If you are thinking about having an abortion, then you need to think again. That's your baby and you can do this. Don't dare let anyone tell you you're not good enough, or not strong enough. This is no way to end up." (Jessica)

Perspective Gatekeeping:

Silencing, Out-Grouping and the Generation of Fear

Censorship of particular views or specific information within the public discourse is a crucial factor in terms of manipulative power. Michel Foucault,[38] a French philosopher who has written extensively on power, sees power as dispersed and pervasive as opposed to embodied in a specific person or thing. He writes extensively on the greater power inherent in discourse control and in particular by the process of discrediting and denying one set of valid statements in order to establish an alternate set of statements as fact.

When control is exerted over not only what can or should be said, but also how or whether particular information is appropriately disseminated, the knowledge and views of people are both restricted and manipulated. Perspective Gatekeeping includes not just censoring information and people out of the discourse through Silencing and Omission, but actively Out-Grouping and Discrediting Dissidents while promoting one's own Experts.

---

38 Foucault, M. (1980). Truth and Power. In C. Gordon (ed.) *Power/Knowledge. Selected Interviews and Other Writings by Michel Foucault, 1972-1977*, Brighton: Havester, 109-133.

Representations of Dissidents as not caring about women, only interested in impeding women's rights, and of misleading and abusing women are replete across the discourse. While declaring one's position as either an Adherent or Dissident is often demanded, the reasons why some may not choose to do this become obvious when such declarations are used as a tool to discredit them. Adherents make it very public that only Adherents can responsibly hold any position of authority if such a position may in any way involve discussions of or decisions about abortion.

This was apparent when Tanya Davies, who self-identified as pro-life, was appointed as the Minister for Women in New South Wales. There was outrage that the new Minister was considered able to represent all women, with clear statements that only 'pro-choice' women could be trusted with such a position:

It is disappointing that the new minister has made her own private views on abortion known so soon.[39] This criticism of the Minister also typifies the contradictions within the discourse; one that demands a declaration, and in this case is then critical when it comes.

The process of emphasising '*our good things and their bad things*' or '*othering*' is a manipulative discourse strategy identified by a range of researchers.[40,41,42] In the article above, many erroneous statements are made about the presumed position of the Minister based on her identification as pro-life. Note that

---

39 Noyes, J. (31 Jan 2017). The Women of NSW Deserve Better Than a Minister Who is 'Personally Pro-Life.' *The Sydney Morning Herald.* https://www.smh.com.au/lifestyle/the-women-of-nsw-deserve-better-than-a-minister-who-is-personally-prolife-20170131-gu1wyr.html
40 van Dijk, Critical Discourse Analysis.
41 Jensen, S. (2011). Othering, Identity Formation and Agency. *Qualitative Studies*, 2(2):63-78.
42 Johnson, J., Bottorff, J., Browne, A., Grewal, S., Hilton, B., and Clarke, H. (2004). Othering and Being Othered in the Context of Health Care Services. *Health Communication*, 16(2):255-271.

Adherents also use their power to re-identify the Minister by their own preferred term of 'anti-choice,' going on to accuse the pro-life positioning as seeking to "control women's reproductive choices through punishment." While offering no clarity as to what such "punishment" consists of, one presumes the 'pro-choice' position sees the support of women in continuation of a pregnancy, and subsequent birth, as punishment.

Discrediting of Dissidents is an important strategy for Adherents as it helps create a discourse that immediately signals that pro-life is essentially bad without ever having to define what is actually bad about it. Adherents will actively discredit any person, whether politician, doctor, counsellor, or even women who express distress about their abortions.

However, this is only one part of Perspective Gatekeeping. The other side is the active promotion of stories and information that normalise or even celebrate abortion.

Shout Your Abortion
(as long as you Toe the Line)

While Adherents have established a range of strategies for normalising and even appearing to celebrate abortion (for example the Shout Your Abortion or End the Stigma campaigns), it is only Adherent women from whom they want to hear. Out-Grouping of women who share their negative experiences of abortion is used as a strategy to both silence and demean them, and is usually accompanied by questioning their motives or even their mental health.

"Shout Your Abortion" was coined as a celebratory announcement of Adherents in an effort to both normalise abortion and give voice to women who had experienced them. Originating in the United States, it quickly became a popular hashtag on social media there and in Australia. The huge headline on the website states, "Our stories are ours to tell," and is described as:

> *"..a decentralized network of individuals talking about abortion on our own terms and creating space for others to do the same. Abortion is normal. Our stories are ours to tell. This is not a debate."*

During this campaign, an Australian woman, Madeleine, shared her story of abortion in an Online Opinion in an article entitled "Choosing abortion is the greatest regret of my life."[43] She shared about the pressures she experienced, and the lack of support she felt for any other option but abortion. She describes the silence of those around her and the platitudes of support:

> *"My GP assumed I would get an abortion so we just discussed how I would go about that. My boyfriend and my family didn't know what to say, so they didn't say much at all…"*

> *"… the people around me in large part stayed silent, except to tell me that they would support me whatever I did. So I [sic] left alone to make this decision."*

..and recalls that nobody prepared her for the possibility that

> *"..when I woke up with relief that this could be replaced with a gnawing hollow regret that would dog me for years."*

It is a highly personal story in which no accusations or judgements are directed toward others who make abortion decisions but reflects her own regret and grief. While there were some supportive comments among the dozens that followed the article, there were also the usual demeaning and dismissive comments:

> *"How dare you try and load your guilt trip on others?"*

> *"If you feel so strongly [that abortion was wrong for you] go adopt an unwanted baby. Rather than spread your propaganda/BS here."*

---

43 Weidemann, M. (18 Oct 2018). Choosing Abortion is the Greatest Regret of My Life. *Online Opinion.* https://www.onlineopinion.com.au/view.asp?article=19994

> *"Perhaps her life has not gone well, and she now glorifies what might have been if she had that baby. Perhaps she suddenly got religion, and that changed her attitude."*

The author is then 'outed' as someone who gave a similarly worded speech at a pro-life meeting and is then told that it is

> *"..clear that she mistakenly identifies her decision to abortion as the cause of her problem, whereas, in fact, it was not the cause, but the solution."*

Della shared her story of deep regret after a coerced abortion on a social media site which claimed to represent women's reproductive rights. She was accused of lying, manipulating, and of being brainwashed. She was then told to take her 'negative vibe' elsewhere.

> *"Hi, we could post a lot more about you or try to press you to answer the question as to whether you are pro-life, but that would be dedicating far too much space and energy to the negative vibe you are introducing to this space. This is a space trying to give voice to the majority. There are plenty of religiously influenced sites encouraging the guilt-ridden and guilt-tripping minority to spread their shaming message. We would ask you again to please head off there."*

When Adherents only allow abortion to be viewed through a lens of positivity and even celebration, while also espousing that "our stories are ours to tell," we can see why so many women are silent when faced with such hostility.

One practitioner noted this among post-abortive patients:

> *"They'll often say they can't deal with the abortion but in a way that says they think it's their own weakness." (General Practitioner)*

Some women are pre-emptively advised that if they don't "get over it" there is something wrong with them:

> *"I was thinking about how when I went to the clinic a nurse told me that I might feel sad after, but that only women who have some kind of tendency to mental illness will stay sad or get really upset about it. Maybe I was one of the ones who was always going to go a bit crazy anyway." (Lena)*

Others get on with things for a while then find themselves thinking more about the abortion as time goes on. Rachel, too, wonders why she is struggling when so many other women don't:

> *"Right after the abortion, I was fine with it, but the more time goes by, the more I am not fine with it. I also know that so many girls get abortions and get along fine. Which makes me wonder what's wrong with me for still crying about it."*

In 2012, a prominent Adherent Expert headed a campaign called End the Stigma[44] which involved pledging support to normalise abortion and end shaming. She refers to people who share anything perceived to threaten abortion as "shame stokers" and claims they are the reason women feel shame about abortion.[45] Bizarrely she also says:

> *"We actually aren't born feeling ashamed of anything. We're not ashamed of our nakedness, we're*

---

44 http://www.september28.org/reproductive-choice-australia/
45 Cannold, L. (2012). I had an abortion… or maybe I didn't. *TEDx Canberra. Speakola.* https://speakola.com/ideas/leslie-cannold-abortion-stigma-tedx-2012

> *not ashamed of our bodily functions, our sexual*
> *desires, our reproduction or abortion."*

Attempting to normalise that which is not a natural biological function, by equating it to functions or aspects that are natural, or by describing it as something on which newborn babies have a perspective, speaks volumes about how disconnected Adherents can be from the reality of such an experience.

She goes on to talk about her view that silence is one aspect that leads to shame and that "shame stokers" are responsible for women remaining silent. Yet considering Madeleine's heartfelt and tragic story of abortion regret above, we can clearly see why women stay silent and it isn't due to shame from Dissidents.

The End the Stigma campaign includes public dancing events by participants wearing Tshirts reading "Abortion. A fact of life. Let's end the stigma."[46] My response to this article pointed out the fact that those who experience abortion negatively also feel silenced and need a voice. This was quickly targeted for Out-Grouping by the Expert. Labelled an "anti-choice activist," the writer invites people to google my own contributions to the discourse, stating:

> *"Debbie is a great example of why the majority*
> *needs to recognise shame-stoking for the damage it*
> *does. Don't feed the trolls."*

I was also described as wanting to "exploit women who experience regret about a terminated pregnancy" and "wanting to perpetuate the stigma of abortion" by the establishment of a website offering regretful women a platform for their stories.[47] For many women contributing to that website, it is the first time they have

---

46 Cannold, L. (18 Sep 2012). Abortion Shaming: What the law does and doesn't do. *Right Now: Human Rights in Australia.* http://rightnow.org.au/opinion-3/abortion-shaming-what-the-law-does-and-doesn%e2%80%99t-do/#disqus_thread
47 http://iregretmyabortion.org.au/

openly spoken about their abortions, even anonymously. The censorship of their stories from the mainstream magnifies their sense that there may be something intrinsically wrong with how they feel. Caroline's experience is common:

> *"I'm so sick of being told how I should or shouldn't feel about my abortion. I remember being told by the clinic that I might feel a bit teary for a week or two but that would be normal; then I'd just be relieved like everyone else. When I rang them six months later because I was STILL teary, they said that was unusual and wouldn't be from the abortion, making me feel like there was something so wrong with me."*

When women like Caroline don't have a positive experience, it may be difficult not only for them to seek help to work through the complexity of their feelings, but also potentially challenging for professionals to develop skills to most effectively help them.

Many professionals are able to identify clients who had experienced abortion negatively, but they often felt ill-equipped to help them. Some also weren't sure that anyone else could either.

> *"There's so few people around that can be trusted to let a woman go through the experience of her grief and her healing." (General Practitioner)*

> *"Some women I'd seen had already been told that their grief was abnormal, that it meant there was some deficit in their coping ability, that it wasn't to do with the abortion itself, after which most women feel relief and just get on with things." (Psychologist)*

46

"There's no question that the woman is suffering, but the system doesn't allow any way for that feedback so that her suffering can be known." (Nurse)

When campaigns such as End the Stigma or Shout Your Abortion are in the mainstream, but the stories of all women are not included, those women who are suffering are even further marginalised. It is not uncommon to hear women (and men) say that their negative emotional experiences have been dismissed as being irrelevant, fabricated, the result of religious brainwashing, or exposure to pro-life propaganda. This likely adds to the isolation that women who are suffering may experience. Many women believe it is just them and wonder why nobody told them:

"I am so confused by how I am feeling. I have never heard of anyone ever not being happy with an abortion. Why didn't I know how big this was?" (Emily)

Adherent women too are often shocked at the discovery that they don't feel like celebrating after an abortion. Felicity had worked in the family violence sector and had often assisted women in gaining access to abortion, believing strongly that it was a right and that it was generally a good thing. Following her own abortion, she didn't think too much about it until her sister was expecting a baby. While out shopping for baby clothes she suddenly experienced a major panic attack, something she had never had before.

"Do I regret my abortion? Absolutely. Would I have made a different decision? Probably not... because I had NO idea this was possible... NO idea that I would even think about it again, let alone that I would feel so overwhelmed with an indefinable

*sorrow in the middle of a Target store that I would
panic." (Felicity)*

These are the stories that Adherents keep hidden, while
actively promoting perceived benefits, dancing and celebrations,
seeking to not only normalise but to glorify a procedure that for
many, even when not regretted, is a traumatic decision and event.
One woman comments on an End the Stigma article:

> *"Whatever, even if I've had an abortion, I'm defi-
> nitely not going to be fucking dancing about it."[48]*

Heather contacted me at the time of the End the Stigma campaign, distressed and wondering where she could go for help:

> *"What is wrong with these people? Even if they want
> women to feel better about abortions, how dare they
> trivialise what happened to me. It isn't something
> I wanted. I wish I didn't have to do it. Don't they
> see they are making me and probably every other
> bloody woman like me just feel worse." (Heather)*

For all the Heathers: no, they don't see. Sadly, even if they do
see it, it seems they don't care. The priority is that the right to
abortion always be there.

---

48 Comment on Cannold, Abortion Shaming.

"There is not something wrong with me for feel-ing sad about the abortion, or even feeling bloody angry like I seem to do a lot more now. I went to the clinic expecting to talk things through, but they had no information for me about what else I could do.

They also talked about how every week I waited it would get more expensive. I didn't even know what I wanted. How can you know when everything feels like your life is falling apart?" (Caroline)

White Ribbon
A Story of Organisational Suicide

It isn't just individuals who incur the wrath of Adherents if they fail to toe the line. Entire organisations can be brought down almost overnight, with people losing their jobs and reputations and services scrambling for damage control. A typical example of organisational Discrediting played out in the media in 2018 when a previously Adherent organisation was Out-Grouped and Discredited for failing to toe the line.

The White Ribbon campaign has international roots as an organisation campaigning against violence against women. The organisation gained momentum in Australia in 2004 and became well known for its celebrity endorsements and national campaigns. In July 2016, Mark Robinson, a Queensland Member of Parliament, joined in the public endorsement of the White Ribbon campaign, posting his support on social media:[49]

> *"As a White Ribbon man, I have pledged to not*
> *ignore DV against women but to stand up against it.*
> *Another reason why I can't support the Pyne-Labor*

---

49 AAP (20 Jul 2016). White Ribbon Rejects Queensland MP Mark Robinson's Link. *Brisbane Times.* https://www.brisbanetimes.com.au/national/queensland/white-ribbon-rejects-queensland-mp-mark-robinsons-link-20160720-gq9k1d.html

> *Abortion Bill as it removes protections for women*
> *against violent partners who are forcing them to*
> *abort the babies they want to keep."*

Mark was at the same time also declaring his strong opposition to political attempts to decriminalise abortion in Queensland. For this reason, White Ribbon quickly distanced themselves from Robinson:

> *"White Ribbon is aware that Queensland MP Mark*
> *Robinson is referencing White Ribbon in his social*
> *media campaigning against a bill to decriminalise*
> *abortion in that state's parliament. We want to reas-*
> *sure our supporters that White Ribbon advocates*
> *for a woman's right to choose. It is a fundamental*
> *human right. Mark Robinson is not and never has*
> *been a White Ribbon Ambassador. He refers to him-*
> *self as a "White Ribbon man," but any man associ-*
> *ated with us should support a woman's right to have*
> *choice over the decisions that relate to her body and*
> *reproductive rights, especially if she is a victim of*
> *violence."*

Prior to that time, there had been no overt public indication of White Ribbon holding any position on abortion. In February of 2017, with the assistance of one of Australia's most active abortion advocacy organisations, Children by Choice, White Ribbon announced a new position statement in support of abortion. In part it stated that abortion is a fundamental human right and included statements advocating for total decriminalisation of abortion throughout the entirety of pregnancy and at no cost to the woman. Citing misinformation about community support for abortion, and health risks to women without greater abortion access, their compliance in toeing the line brought forth significant praise from Adherents.

In that same year, a motion was put forward in Federal parliament to challenge the position of White Ribbon on this issue in light of receiving federal funding. While the motion was defeated, it drew an Alarmist and misleading response from one Senator who shouted,

> *"You bunch of misogynistic... This is about rape victims having access to safe and legal abortion. That's what you just voted against."*[50]

With less than one percent of abortions being undertaken as a result of rape, and then mostly in the first trimester of pregnancy, abortion availability during the entirety of pregnancy for all women is clearly not about rape victims.

In October 2018, White Ribbon made a decision to consult with their stakeholders on their position on abortion, taking down their position statement and claiming that until such consultation took place, they were taking an "agnostic" position on the issue. The then CEO, Tracey McLeod Howe, stated that some supporters had objected to White Ribbon taking a political position on an issue without consultation.

Once the removal of the abortion position statement was discovered, the backlash from Adherents was both swift and hostile with the move being described in Alarmist terms across social media as a "scandal," "pretty horrific," "most concerning," and that it "sends a dangerous message to women."[51] Within hours, organisations were announcing their withdrawal of support for

---

50 Ireland, J. (17 Nov 2017). Coalition senators defy government position to cross the floor over Cory Bernardi anti-abortion ploy. *The Sydney Morning Herald.* https://www.smh.com.au/politics/federal/coalition-senators-defy-government-position-to-cross-the-floor-over-cory-bernardi-antiabortion-ploy-20171116 gzmoey.html
51 Price, J. (22 Oct 2018). It's Time to Shut the White Ribbon Campaign Down. *Sydney Morning Herald.* https://www.smh.com.au/opinion/it-s-time-to-shut-the-white-ribbon-campaign-down-20181021-p50b33.html

White Ribbon, and there were calls for the organisation to be closed down.

In the midst of this, McLeod Howe tried desperately to maintain her status as an Adherent by statements of regret for removing the position statement from the website and protestations that she had paid for women's abortions in the past, and that she supported women's right to access abortion.[52] However, Adherent feminists talked about her as having been a "disappointing choice" for CEO and argued that the organisation had never been truly supportive of women and according to one Expert was obviously just "an agent of patriarchy:"

> *"Apparently White Ribbon have withdrawn their support for reproductive rights. In that case they are no longer a pro-women organisation but an agent of patriarchy. Without control of our bodies, there is no liberty."[53]*

Caro had previously lauded the organisation as both effective in its work and courageous in taking a stance on abortion, going so far as to equate them to Marie Stopes, one of Australia's largest abortion providers:[54]

> *"Like Marie Stopes, White Ribbon have identified that access to legal and affordable abortion is an important part of women's safety."*

52Tracy McLeod says she was wrong to remove the statements but denies she buckled to pressure from religious groups. Henriques-Gomes, L. (19 Oct 2018). White Ribbon Australia reinstates statements backing reproductive rights on website. *The Guardian.* https://www.theguardian.com/australia-news/2018/oct/19/white-ribbon-australia-reinstates-statements-backing-reproductive-rights-on-website
53 Caro, J. (Twitter) (October 19, 2018). Cited in Henriques-Gomes, White Ribbon Australia reinstates statements.
54 Caro, J. (23 Nov 2017). Two Heated Issues Down, One to Go: We Need to Talk About Abortion. *ABC News.* http://www.abc.net.au/news/2017-11-23/jane-caro-abortion-rights-my-choice-marie-stopes-white-ribbon/9181742

It was also suggested by one Expert academic that

> *"We should be deeply concerned that the chief executive of an organisation purporting to be about stopping violence against women thinking she needs to consult on reproductive rights with her stakeholders."*[55]

In spite of her frantic backpedalling and profuse apologies, less than a month later it was announced that McLeod Howe had left her position and the previous CEO reinstated, as was White Ribbon's policy on abortion.

As an organisation, White Ribbon was not established for the purpose of promoting or engaging in discussions about reproductive rights, and apart from the one position statement, their primary work had nothing to do with the issue. Yet when this one issue was flagged for further consultation with stakeholders, the entire organisational work and the CEO were personally and professionally Discredited. This demonstrates the rapid Alarmist responses from Adherents to any perceived dissent and the way in which no matter how effectively one works to toe the line, not a single waver from the line is tolerated or can be forgiven. It also demonstrates the power of social media as significant in surveillance and control of dissent.

---

55 Price, It's Time to Shut the White Ribbon Campaign Down.

"On the one hand I really wanted my baby. On the other, I knew my partner would hate me for keeping it. I also didn't want him to hate my baby. I didn't ever want to have to explain to my precious child that his or her father didn't want him or her. I had in my hands the life of my child, my own life, my boyfriend's life and our families. It wasn't a decision that affected only me." (Joni)

Academic Censoring

One expects that education in universities and research should remain out of reach of ideological concerns so that people are free to question and discover without censorship. Unfortunately, this is no longer the case, particularly on this very sensitive issue, but disturbingly in a growing number of other controversial subject areas as well.

In universities across Australia, students have battled to establish pro-life groups with a view to both educating about issues women face during pregnancy and parenting, and establishing services to support them. They have faced fierce opposition that attempts to both ban their existence and disrupt their activities, even when such activities are devoted to ensuring supports for pregnant and parenting students.

When the University of Tasmania LifeChoice group was established with the mission to,

> *"promote the dignity of human life from conception*
> *to natural death, through reasonable and informed*
> *discussion on the issues of abortion and euthanasia*
> *in Australian Society."*[56]

..a representative of the University's Women's Collective

---

56 https://lifechoice.org.au/

responded,

> *"Students have the right to feeling safe on campus and an education free from harassment and discrimination. The affiliation and presence of 'LifeChoice' on campus compromises this."*[57]

A group with the same mission attempted to establish at a Western Australian university with swift action by pro-choice groups describing it as a "divisive anti-abortion organisation."[58] Arguing that the establishment of such a group was distressing, and that women don't need to be lectured about their decisions, they went on to say that "these matters are best placed with unbiased counsellors or medical professionals."

Of course, "unbiased" is in the eye of the ideology. With so many who are concerned about abortion becoming too afraid to speak, and those who toe the line unprepared to tell the truth for fear of risking reputation and livelihoods, women are left with only themselves, and a discourse that provides little if any accessible accurate information.

On invitation by pro-life groups, I've spoken at a few university events. On arriving on one occasion, flyers promoting the event had been defaced with pictures of coat hangers and dripping blood and a range of derogatory insults. Another event had to be moved to an off-campus location due to threats of disruption. On arrival at the off-campus location around 30 students were on the sidewalk screaming profanity into megaphones and drawing graphic depictions of blood and coat hangers on the sidewalk.

---

57 Grant, S. (n.d.). Remove Ant-Abortion Group @ UTAS (petition). https://www.megaphone.org.au/petitions/remove-anti-abortion-group-from-tuu?fbclid=IwAR3z5Fdkh1n-wLJxcAz1_pXrlYawYycBjOfyNMdNtSNcVC5DNeB4IvEY1QO8
58 Hiatt, B. (17 Apr 2018). Notre Dame University Students Reject Anti-Abortion Organisation, Life Choice Australia. *The West Australian*, https://thewest.com.au/news/education/notre-dame-university-students-reject-anti-abortion-organisation-lifechoice-australia-ng-b88802003z

None seemed concerned that passers-by, including children, may have been distressed by their antics and drawings.

On both occasions, the topic of the event was geared toward ways in which universities could develop supportive educational opportunities for pregnant and parenting students so that they did not experience abortion as their only option for continuing education. Adherent students perceived this as an anti-abortion activity.

On another occasion at a university speaking engagement, a group of four young women who had been sitting in the front rows rolling their eyes and giggling through much of my talk ran straight up to me as soon as I'd finished speaking. *"We're with the women's collective here on campus and we're pro-choice,"* one said with seeming delight. My reply was, *"Congratulations, what is your campus doing to ensure pregnant and parenting students can choose to continue their educations?"*

It was as though they had prepared a speech and I hadn't said my lines correctly when they all looked a little confused and quizzical. *"Well, nothing,"* one replied, *"we're here to make sure they can get abortions."* One of their group piped up and said, *"Why aren't we doing anything about that?"* (supporting pregnant and parenting students). An interesting conversation ensued about what constituted "choice" with me repeating much of what I'd just presented that had previously escaped their attention. This is typical behaviour of Adherent groups of young people in universities. They are generally the manipulated, with no idea that what they espouse may be flawed or ill-considered, or that the alternatives are worthy of attention.

It isn't surprising that so many lack a fuller perspective of reproductive health issues when it is challenging to get research on adverse effects of abortion published and when researchers who undertake this task are Discredited.

Even Adherent researchers courageous enough to undertake research on abortion can often experience significant hurdles in trying to get their research published. One such researcher, David Fergusson, a self-proclaimed atheist and pro-choice advocate who is widely published in other topical areas, stated that he was rejected by four journals before finally having his article published because it found a significantly increased mental health risk in women following abortion.[59]

> *"We expected to find no evidence of harmful effects of abortion. But we found the opposite.*
>
> *The paper was declined by a number of journals, he suspects because of the controversial nature of the topic. "We went to four journals, which is very unusual for us—we normally get accepted the first time."*
>
> *He knew that by publishing the paper, he and the group would be throwing themselves into a vicious political arena, and their science would be claimed as "proof" of a certain ideology by one side, and damned by the other."[60]*

Fergusson was also the subject of a social media discussion where he was labelled a "bad researcher" and that he had been entirely "debunked." No distinction was made between the research he undertook to find increased mental health risks from abortion and his other research.

One practitioner I spoke to was shocked by the numbers of women he had seen who were struggling after abortion and

---

59 Fergusson, D., Horwood, L. and Ridder, E. (2006). Abortion in Young Women and Subsequent Mental Health. *Journal of Child Psychology and Psychiatry*, 47(1):16-24.
60 Hill, R. (5 Jan 2006). Abortion Researcher Confounded by Study. New Zealand Herald. https://www.nzherald.co.nz/nz/abortion-researcher-confounded-by-study/

considered publishing some case studies from his practice. He lamented his decision not to as he thought the information was very important, but said,

> *"I knew if I took that step, my career path was over."*

When information in education, research, and literature on adverse impacts of abortion is so restricted and what little does manage to slip through the censorship net is Discredited, it is no surprise that women who seek support often find it unavailable.

> *"I let everyone tell me how bad it would be to have a less than perfect baby. I did everything I knew how to do. I spoke to everyone I knew to speak to. They all had nothing but bad news.*
>
> *I remember laying in that bed while one nurse put a drip in my arm, staring at another nurse, willing her to tell me there was another way. When she came over to me I thought she must have heard my thoughts... I had hope... I almost pulled my arm away. Then she looked at me and said, "It's okay, we don't judge you here." (Libby, abortion at 24 weeks)*

"For the sake of a bit of embarrassment about being pregnant, an interruption to what I considered to be my very important life, I had dumped that baby like trash. And other people helped me do it, just like I have helped my friends.

I was too embarrassed to even tell my best friend I'd had such an irresponsible accident as to fall pregnant. But the clinic I went to made it oh so easy... A little group info session where we heard that we'll all feel relieved and be able to go home as though nothing had happened... where we were told the procedure was simple with no lasting effects...

And I believed it all, even afterwards... for three and half years, to be exact. Until the night I felt this baby kicking under my ribs.

I've been advocating for choice for women my entire adult life. I've taken two friends to abortion clinics. I've written letters to the editor berating pro-lifers for being judgemental, religious zealots who care nothing for women. Yet, in this moment, everything changed. I realised that the only difference between this baby and the one I so denied was nothing at all, nothing at all except my own shame and self-importance three years ago." (Helen)

Community Manipulation

How Adherents Claim Majority Support

Majority support for abortion is claimed by Adherents as a reason for censoring and shutting down any debate on the issue. It has been effectively used as a strategy to change abortion legislation which has resulted in even greater restrictions on essential information for women. It infringes on the rights of doctors and those who would seek to provide support to women considering abortion. Given what you now know about the way in which people are recruited to the cause of abortion rights and the restriction of information, it should come as no surprise to learn that community surveys on abortion are often completely unreliable.

While addressing the practical aspects of community attitude surveys, this chapter will expand on some of the theory about why people are so prepared to conform and to simply accept what is told to them. Theories include Festinger's (1962) Theory of Cognitive Dissonance, Proctor's (2008) Theory of Agnotology, and Noelle-Neumann's (1974) concept of the Spiral of Silence. Each of these contributes to explanations as to why community attitude surveys are unlikely to be a reliable reflection of the reality of public opinion in the setting of Alarmist Gatekeeping.

We know that one way in which the power of the Dominant Discourse is maintained and perpetuated is by recruitment to a 'common' cause. This is made all the more powerful by suggestions that the majority of people support the cause, therefore if you don't you belong in the Out-Group. People who support abortion are "good" and people who don't are "bad." This positive self-representation and negative "other" representation as an aspect of Out-Grouping is a typical strategy occurring within manipulative discourses.[61] The idea that "most people agree" applies a psychological pressure to conform that can be powerful enough to override one's personal values even on an issue of such importance as abortion.[62]

As is the case with many issues, people often do not give a tremendous amount of thought to something that doesn't directly impact them. This leaves most knowledge being absorbed passively by the Discourse to which people are exposed.

Maintaining the Ignorance

Proctor's research into ignorance, or what he terms Agnotology, holds some relevance for the manipulative patterns identified in Alarmist Gatekeeping.[63] Of particular interest are his descriptions of different types of ignorance, how these apply to those affected by the Discourse, and how they are utilised to further the aims of the Discourse.

Proctor describes three types of ignorance:
1. Native state, which describes a lack of knowing which is remedied by new information and knowledge. We most commonly consider ignorance in this way.

---

61 van Dijk, Discourse and Manipulation.
62 Noelle-Neumann, E. (1974). The Spiral of Silence: A Theory of Public Opinion. *The Journal of Communication,* 24(2):43-51.
63 Proctor, R. (2008). *Agnotology: The Making and Unmaking of Ignorance.* Stanford University Press.

2. Ignorance as a selective choice or passive construct, which occurs as a result of the inability to attend to all things and choosing which to attend to: "a way of seeing is also a way of not seeing—a focus on object A involves a neglect of object B."

Many people base at least a portion of their knowledge of abortion or other controversial or polarising issues on what they learn from the media, and on what they believe to be the most popular opinion.[64] Abortion is an uncomfortable subject for many, so unless there is some reason for them to seek out information, people may be more likely to choose to believe the Dominant Messaging without question.

3. Ignorance as a strategic ploy or active construct, whereby there is an active intention to control what people know, and how they know it. This is achieved by means of creating doubt and disseminating misinformation.

The power of ignorance as a strategic ploy is demonstrated in Alarmist Gatekeeping through information restriction and censorship. When factual knowledge threatens to override ignorance, strategies of Discrediting and Out-Grouping ensure the perpetuation of ignorance for the majority.

Proctor uses the tobacco industry as an example of constructed ignorance. Advocates of cigarette smoking actively promoted the virtues of cigarette smoking while actively creating doubt about harms. On the issue of abortion, the benefits may be promoted in negative terms such as "saving women from dying" or more positively framed, "to ensure equality for women."

On a social level of manipulation, van Dijk goes so far as to suggest those who succumb to such manipulation could be considered victims, with victims defined as those who lack the

64 Hayes, A. (2017). Exploring the Forms of Self-Censorship: On the Spiral of Silence and Use of Opinion Expression Avoidance Strategies, *Journal of Communication*, 57:785-802.

resources to "resist, detect or avoid manipulation."[65] He suggests four contextual criteria for this to occur:

1. Incomplete or lack of relevant knowledge—so that no counter-arguments can be formulated against false, incomplete, or biased assertions.
2. Fundamental norms, values, and ideologies that cannot be denied or ignored.
3. Strong emotions, traumas, etc. that make people vulnerable.
4. Social positions, professions, status etc. that induce people into tending to accept the discourse, arguments etc. of elite persons, groups or organisations.

Each of these is seen within Alarmist Gatekeeping on abortion.

1. Incomplete or lack of relevant knowledge: When the Dominant Discourse supports only a single acceptable perspective on abortion that dominates educational settings and academic articles while Discrediting alternate views, it can be challenging to gain factual knowledge.
2. Fundamental norms: The single perspective on abortion has become so ingrained that the majority of people (Incognisants) have internalised it as truth and are reluctant to question it, given the prevalence of Out-Grouping that is witnessed.
3. Strong emotions, traumas, etc.: The issue of abortion raises the emotional level for many people whether because they disagree with the Dominant Discoursing, have experienced abortion, or have ambivalent feelings about the issue.
4. Social Positions: Adherent 'Experts' are generally those imbued as wiser, more educated, and with status.

---

65 van Dijk, Discourse and Manipulation.

From a broader community level, it can be seen how the combination of properties of Alarmist Recruitment and Perspective Gatekeeping work together to elicit community compliance with the Dominant Discourse.

Cognitive Dissonance and the Spiral of Silence

The widespread prevalence of the Dominant perspective combined with many of the above criteria are powerful in themselves. However, there are more micro, individual considerations that mean people are more likely to accept the Dominant view. The Alarmist Gatekeeping messaging is pervasive, consistent, and therefore more familiar.[66] An alternate view may create discomfort which people want to avoid.[67,68]

Leon Festinger's theory of Cognitive Dissonance may provide some explanation for the way in which the minds of people are easily dissuaded from uncomfortable facts about abortion. Festinger proposed that if two cognitions seem equally important, but are logically inconsistent or contradictory, discomfort arises. When this dissonance occurs, the person either changes their behaviour or seeks some information to either confirm one of the cognitions or reduce or eliminate the significance of the other. Cassagrande[69] discusses this point:

> *"Most importantly, research has clearly shown that people want to avoid cognitive dissonance very much and are therefore willing to embrace abstract rhetoric of their leaders, even when there are obvious contradictions, or their leaders are involving*

66 Moons, Mackie, and Garcie-Marques, The Impact of Repetition-Induced Familiarity.
67 Festinger, L. (1962). *A Theory of Cognitive Dissonance,* Stanford University Press.
68 Newby-Clark, I. R., McGregor, I., and Zanna, M. P. (2002). Thinking and Caring About Cognitive Inconsistency: When and for Whom Does Attitudinal Ambivalence Feel Uncomfortable? *Journal of Personality and Social Psychology, 82*(2):157–166.
69 Cassagrande, D. (2004). *Power and the Rhetorical Manipulation of Cognitive Dissonance*, Paper delivered at the Presidential session of the Annual Meeting of the American Anthropological Association. December 15-19, Atlanta.

> *ideas that would not be palatable in other contexts.*
> *Leaders, in turn, discourage people from critically*
> *examining details or considering potential contra-*
> *dictions by steering the public discourse away from*
> *potential inconsistencies."*

Consider the fact that late-term abortions occur at a rate of six a week, every week, in one state alone in Australia, and that around half of these are on healthy babies. For many this information is horrifying, or at least uncomfortable. Believing it requires dealing with that discomfort or maybe even acting on it. It is much simpler and safer to fall back on relying on the Experts who will be quick to refute such facts and make sure you understand that those who espouse them are "bad" people.

Noelle-Neumann talks about the social control of public opinion of value-laden issues. She asserts that the power of public control of public opinion stems from the willingness of people to threaten to socially isolate those who dissent from the required view, and the individual's fear of isolation. This doesn't mean that all people come to agree with the Dominant view, but that fewer people have the courage to speak their disagreement and alternate views in order to avoid being isolated. Noelle-Neumann also suggests some cognitive processes a person might undertake in order to decide when they might risk isolation:

> *"...by observing his social environment, by assess-*
> *ing the distribution of opinions for and against his*
> *ideas, but above all by evaluating the strength (com-*
> *mitment), the urgency, and the chances of success of*
> *certain proposals and viewpoints."[70]*

This process may be also be considered a process of conformity as described by Cialdini and Goldstein (2004) in their review of

70 Noelle-Neumann, The Spiral of Silence.

research on social influence. Conformity is a process whereby the individual matches their own behaviour or responses to what they see others doing as a means of belonging. These processes add to the power of manipulation that Alarmist Gatekeeping has; it drives legislation which further reinforces the view of majority public opinion.

Through just this one snapshot of social and psychological processes, we can see how easy it can be to deceive the majority or at least ensure they toe the line through Alarmist Gatekeeping. We don't want to feel uncomfortable. We don't want to be different. We want to belong. This has significant impacts on how we think and how we might respond to surveys on abortion.

"I'm absolutely pro-choice and have marched for women's reproductive rights. It's so important that we don't go backwards on this issue. Of course there is no excuse for abortion after twelve weeks, unless the woman or baby is going to die or really suffer of course. But up to then, women need abortions and should be able to get them." (Jacquie)

Recruiting You to "Yes"

Community attitudes on important issues can significantly influence legislative action. One would think that ensuring reliability of such information would be a priority. However, when Alarmist Gatekeeping is at work, there are compelling reasons for ensuring general community agreement with the Dominant Messaging, and easy ways to ensure this occurs. It begins by controlling the information to which people have access and on which they base their views, followed by ensuring good recruiting questions. For this reason, the majority of surveys of community attitudes toward abortion tend to limit questions to the issue of a woman's right to abortion as opposed to the context of her circumstances.

As part of its task in reporting on decriminalisation legislation in Victoria in 2008, one of the terms of reference was that the Victorian Law Reform Commission (VLRC) was *"to consider and develop law reform options that reflect current community standards."*[71] They identified five published studies as having some rigour, stating that the results therein assisted the commission to "identify points of consensus in what is a highly polarised debate."

---

71 Victorian Law Reform Commission (2008). *Law of Abortion: Final Report 15.* Victorian Law Reform Commission. https://www.lawreform.vic.gov.au/sites/default/files/VLRC_Abortion_Report.pdf

In brief, the surveys relied on were as follows.

The Australian Survey of Social Attitudes, conducted in 2005, asked whether respondents agreed with this statement:

A woman should have the right to choose whether or not she has an abortion.[72]

This is a general statement seeking support for the principle of rights. The majority of the general public, subject to a Discourse that tells them abortion is only (or mostly) accessed for very serious or life-threatening reasons, will say they agree with such a statement and 79% of them did. This is then used to suggest support for all abortion access.

The Australian Election Study question was a little more specific in providing some context.[73] Conducted in 2004, respondents were asked to rate which one of the following statements came closest to their feelings about abortion:

a. Women should be able to obtain an abortion readily when they want one.
b. Abortion should only be allowed in special circumstances.
c. Abortion should not be allowed under any circumstances.
d. Don't know.

In contrast to the first survey only 54% of people agreed that abortion should be "readily available" on demand, with 35% selecting only in special circumstances.

72 Wilson, S., Gibson, R., Denemark, D. and Western, M. (eds.) (2005) *Australian Social Attitudes: The First Report.* UNSW Press, Sydney.
73 Bean, C., McAllister, I., Gibson, R., Gow, D. (2005). *Australian Election Study 2004.* Australian National University.

The Southern Cross Bioethics Institute Survey was commissioned in 2004 and asked for "personal opinions, that is, how you feel personally on the issue,"[74]
'whether women should have unrestricted access to abortion on demand, no matter what the circumstance.'

Response options ranged from "Strongly Agree" through to "Strongly Disagree" and "Undecided" with 62% of respondents somewhat or strongly in agreement. Respondents were also asked whether they believed there are too many abortions in Australia; 61% agreed that there were, highlighting the often conflictual feelings that people have on the issue. When asked if there was a way to reduce abortion numbers while still giving women the right to freely choose, 88% believed this would be a good thing.

The Marie Stopes International Survey in 2003 included 6593 respondents who had experienced an unplanned pregnancy. They were asked for their responses to three questions based on their current view and their view "at the time of your unplanned pregnancy:"[75]

a. Women should be able to obtain an abortion readily when they want one.
b. Abortion should be allowed only in special circumstances.
c. Abortion should not be allowed in any circumstances.

There was not a significant difference between views at the time

74 Fleming, J. and Tonti-Filippini, N. (eds), (2007) *Common Ground? Seeking an Australian Consensus on Abortion and Sex Education*. St Pauls Press.
75 Marie Stopes (2006). *Women, Contraception, and Unplanned Pregnancy*. https://www.mariestopes.org.au/wp-content/uploads/Real-Choices-Key-Findings.pdf

of an unplanned pregnancy and current views with 60% choosing
option A and 30% option B.

The Australian Federation of Right to Life Associations Survey
conducted in 2005 over two stages was much more specific,
providing a greater context within questions:[76]

In Stage 1, two questions elicited respondents' general views
on abortion:

> Do you support abortion for any reason whatsoever, that is,
> abortion on demand?

> Do you support abortion for non-medical, that is, for finan-
> cial or social reasons?

In Stage 2 there were two questions about stages of pregnancy
at which abortion should be allowed:

Up to what stage of pregnancy would you allow abortion?

> 1. At any time up to 13 weeks, that is 3 months
> 2. At any time up to 20 weeks, that is half-way through
> pregnancy
> 3. At any time during pregnancy up to birth
> 4. Not at all
> 5. Don't know

Would you allow late-term abortion after 20 weeks of pregnancy for non-medical, that is in cases of financial or emotional
stress? (Yes/No/Don't Know)

Stage 1 respondents demonstrated that 60% supported abortion
on demand, but also that 51% opposed abortion for financial or

---

76 Australian Federation of Right to Life Associations Survey (2005), cited in Victorian
Law Reform Commission, Law of Abortion.

social reasons, whereas 34% of Stage 2 respondents said abortion should not be allowed at all, and 39% said only up to 13 weeks. Of Stage 3 respondents, 82% would not allow abortion after 20 weeks for non-medical reasons, with only 12% saying they would. The strength of this survey was in its specificity of questioning with respondents able to provide their views on more detailed scenarios.

The most interesting aspect of this survey is how it highlights the confusion and conflict that people have between wanting to support "rights" and not being comfortable with abortion in many contexts.

Each of the surveys was deemed by the VLRC to have both strengths and limitations, with strengths including the more nuanced questions of the Australian Federation of Right to Life Associations Survey. Interestingly, the identified strength of the Australian Survey of Social Attitudes included that the survey results were "subject to peer review and published in scholarly journals." No mention is made of whether researchers of the other surveys ever sought publication or were rejected. If this was the case, the challenges of publishing research that is perceived to threaten abortion rights would need to be considered as a factor.

Identified limitations included low response rates, single non-specific questions and survey designs. One of the conclusions of the VLRC was that "a majority of Australians support a woman's right to choose whether to have an abortion."[77] Abortion was subsequently decriminalised in Victoria, allowing abortion on demand to 24 weeks of pregnancy and after that on the approval of two doctors.

The way in which survey results are presented to the public usually entails a misleading exaggeration of support for abortion, while minimising or ignoring any aspects that may be a threat.

---

77 Victorian Law Reform Commission, Law of Abortion.

Adherents frequently recruit support for abortion by statements such as that by the Australian Reproductive Health Alliance:

> *"It is overwhelmingly clear that the majority of Australians support liberal access to abortion."*[78]

However, their own survey results report that the "majority" constitutes only 54.2% with the remaining 45.8% wanting restrictions on access or no access at all. Queensland Adherent organisation Children by Choice use the results of the 2003 Australian Survey of Social Attitudes as a recruitment tool, stating that,

> *"..reliable opinion polling consistently shows that around 80% of Australian adults support a woman's right to choose."*[79]

One study undertaken in Victoria in 2008 and published in a medical journal asked specific questions about abortion at different gestational ages and in different circumstances.[80] The results of the research included that only 6% of respondents believe abortion should be available without restriction in the third trimester, with 48% believing abortion should be illegal regardless of circumstances at this time, and 28% of people believing abortion should be illegal in the second trimester, which is after 12 weeks. Yet the authors concluded that their study shows,

> *"..remarkably strong public support for women being able to access abortion at all stages of pregnancy including after 24 weeks."*

On occasion, media outlets conduct online surveys and publish

---

78 Australian Reproductive Health Alliance (2004). *What do Australians Think About Abortion*, Australian Reproductive Health Alliance.

79 https://www.childrenbychoice.org.au/factsandfigures/attitudestoabortion

80 De Crespigny, L. Wilkinson, D., Douglas, T., Textor, M. and Savulescu, J. (2010). Australian Attitudes to Early and Late Abortion. *The Medical Journal of Australia*, 193(1): 9-12.

results, which are also invariably interpreted as demonstrating majority support for abortion, for example "*only a small minority want more restrictive abortion laws.*"[81] However these often fail to ask more than general questions about rights or restrictions without giving context or making any effort to determine the knowledge base of respondents.

Some researchers have attempted to develop what they deem to be more reliable methods of measuring attitudes on abortion. Taylor and Whitehead[82] developed a survey tool for the measurement of abortion attitudes in 2014 and stated that it and the Hess and Rueb[83] scale developed in 2005 are both reliable and valid for this purpose. However, neither of the developers or published papers make any reference to how to address the knowledge, or accuracy of knowledge, that respondents may have about abortion, nor the pressures that exist within the Discourse to comply with the Dominant position. The possibility that people in the community self-censor in a way similar to practitioners in this study needs to be considered.

None of the research findings on community attitudes accounts for the social and psychological pressures that may exist in the presence of value-laden issues. The knowledge base that members of the community have about abortion and the situations which compel women to seek abortion are also ignored. In the absence of identification or acknowledgment of these factors, the reliability of surveys on this and other value-laden research must be questionable.

---

81   Stayner, G. (24 Nov 2014). Victorian election 2014: Majority support same-sex adoption, fewer restrictions on abortion, Vote Compass reveals. *ABC News.* https://www.abc.net.au/news/2014-11-24/support-for-same-sex-adoption-fewer-restrictions-on-abortion/5912602?nw=0
82 Taylor, M. and Whitehead, G. (2014). The Measurement of Attitudes Toward Abortion. *Modern Psychological Studies,* 20(1):79-86.
83 *Hess,* J. A. and *Rueb,* J. D. (2005). *Attitudes* Toward *Abortion,* Religion, and Party Affiliation Among College Students. *Current Psychology,* 24:24–42.

There are not only social pressures to conform because of the publicly demonstrated risks of Out-Grouping and Discrediting. Internal psychological pressures to belong and not be isolated are also significant. The responses of community attitude surveys are often presented in the media as more supportive of abortion than they actually are, further applying pressure to conform. Surveys are also being used to inform legislators, and the laws created further reinforce the perception of views, creating a perpetuating loop from which few have the courage to dissent.

"My sister had a baby girl five weeks ago, only one week before the date my baby would have been due to be born. Everybody is so happy. She is the first grandchild. She is so beautiful. I held her on the day she was born, felt the softness of her skin and smelt her. I didn't want to stop smelling her. I don't think I've smelt a new baby before. How can they smell so good?

When I got into my car after leaving the hospital, I began to cry, sitting there in the car park, tears just streaming down my face. I couldn't understand it. I just kept crying. I was thankful it was dark so nobody could see me sitting there. Suddenly I was crying so hard, and feeling like I was suffocating and panicking. I opened the car door thinking I needed to get out; I stood up, but I didn't know where to go. That's when it hit me; the smell of that little girl was like something so familiar, something I knew but couldn't remember. Sitting there in that car I realised it was the smell of the baby I wasn't having.

"I aborted my baby, a baby I hadn't thought of as a baby until that moment. It was matter of fact. My boyfriend was married. He didn't want to leave his wife. I didn't want him to leave his children. It was the right thing to do. I didn't tell anyone. I didn't even ask my boyfriend to pay for it. It was easy. I didn't give it a lot of thought, not then, and not even a couple of weeks later when my sister announced her pregnancy. In fact I didn't really think about it again at all.

Now I can't stop. Now I look at my sister's little girl and all I think about is what I did, what I've lost, the smell of her. I am so confused by how I am feeling. I have never heard of anyone ever not being happy with an abortion. Why didn't I know how big this was? I'm not a teenager. I'm educated. I killed my child and I didn't even blink. I haven't cried again since that day in the car-park. I can't afford to. I don't feel anything. I have nowhere to go. I will never forgive myself. "(Karla)

Toeing the Line

Maintaining the Silence

At some point in the continuum between a positive pregnancy test, seeking an abortion and having had an abortion, women may meet with a range of different professionals. It might be their own doctor, a nurse or social worker, the abortion provider or their staff. The power of Alarmist Gatekeeping is demonstrated by the way in which such practitioners self-censor even in the privacy of a one-to-one confidential consultation with a client.

Adherent, Incognisant and Dissident practitioners all self-censor in some way, although for different reasons. All are subject to the Dominant Discourse on abortion along with the rest of us, with the added influences of professional body positions, collegial expectations, and legislative requirements. Thus, while practitioners are vulnerable to the psychological need to conform, legislation is an added element in the decision toward compliance as well.

Fear of reprisals, whether real or perceived, practical, reputational or psychological, can be enough to modify behaviour both in public and in more private settings such as those of a practitioner-client interaction. In Australia, censorship is used with powerful effect when combined with the Discrediting that

81

co-exists with Out-Grouping. The way in which manipulation occurs through censorship is multi-faceted, involving not only the omission of information, but also the Discrediting of information once it becomes public. It is as much a process as it is a range of discrete activities. Curry Jansen provides a comprehensive definition of censorship that encompasses most elements of what this theory proposes in abortion discoursing:[84]

> *"...the term encompasses all socially structured proscriptions or prescriptions which inhibit or prohibit dissemination of ideas, information, images, and other messages through a society's channels of communication whether these obstructions are secured by political, economic, religious or other systems of authority. It includes both overt and covert proscriptions and prescriptions."*

While Incognisants may censor what they say as a way of conforming, Dissidents may do so as a way to avoid Out-Grouping and Discrediting, and some Adherents do so in order to "protect the pro-choice movement."[85] Ludlow describes a hierarchy of abortion stories that have specific intentions ranging from upholding and maintaining abortion rights through to threatening rights.[86] 'Acceptable' stories include those involving the need for abortion in cases of rape, incest, or foetal abnormalities. However a category of 'things we cannot say' includes the existence of grief after abortion and women having multiple abortions.

> *"Self-censorship may also be motivated by the _____ desire to defend and uphold a particular idea, a*

84 Curry Jansen, S. (1988). *Censorship: The Knot That Binds Power and Knowledge.* Oxford University Press, New York, p221.
85 Martin, L., Hassinger J., Debbink M. and Harris, L. (2017). Dangertalk: Voices of Abortion Providers. *Social Science Medicine,* 184:75-83.
86 Ludlow, J. (2008). The Things We Cannot Say: Witnessing the Traumatisation of Abortion in the United States. *WSQ Women's Studies Quarterly,* 36(1):28-41.

*value, dogma, goal, policy, ideology or belief. Indi-
viduals who adhere to a particular view may be
motivated to uphold it even in the face of contra-
dicting information."*[87]

The behaviour that Adherents want to be adopted among practitioners and the general public is that of unquestioningly upholding the principle of abortion rights. One of the explicit aims of
abortion advocacy is the normalisation of abortion in the belief
that this will reduce stigma and increase availability and access
for women.[88,89] Yet research on abortion workers demonstrates
that even in the setting of service provision there exists judgements and stigma toward women that are controlled by toeing
the line.[90,91,92]

Martin and colleagues spoke to people working in abortion
provision about their experiences. One worker says they describe
women having repeat abortions as *"frequent flyers"* and describes
her feelings about that: *"She comes in for #15 abortion. And I just
had a little problem with that."* Others talked about their own
concerns around moral uncertainty: *"I still to this day say to
myself I hope I'm doing the right thing. That never goes away."*

One clinician describes the way in which it is their responsibility to prioritise abortion access above talking about the reality

87 Bar-Tal, D. (2017). Self-Censorship as a Socio-Political-Psychological Phenomenon: Conception and Research. *Advances in Political Psychology,* 38(Suppl.1).

88 Doran, F. and Hornibrook, J. (2015). Barriers around access to abortion experienced by rural women in New South Wales, Australia. *The International Electronic Journal of Rural and Remote Health Research, Education, Practice and Policy*, 16(1):3538.

89 Kumar, A., Hessini, L. and Mitchell, E. (2009). Conceptualising abortion stigma. *Culture, Health and Sexuality*, 11(6):625-639.

90 Lipp, A. (2010). Concealing and Conceding Judgement in Termination of Pregnancy: A Grounded Theory Study. *Journal of Research in Nursing*, 15(4):365-378.

91 Martin, Hassinger, Debbink and Harris, Dangertalk.

92 Newton, D., Bayly, C., McNamee, K., Hardiman, A., Bismark, M., Webster, A. and Keogh, L. (2016). How do women seeking abortion choose between surgical and medical abortion? Perspectives from abortion service providers. *Australian and New Zealand Journal of Obstetrics and Gynaecology,* 56:523-529.

83

of the experience for women:

> *"I'm aware that any bad experience could set us back so much... if... people talk about it and... tell people how bad it is, and how you can get hurt from it. I feel like it's part of my responsibility in some fucked up way to make sure that I help keep abortions going."*

Newton's Australian study[93] found that most providers withhold their professional opinion about the most appropriate abortion method based on a woman's personal risk factors because they

> *"..appeared to have strong desire to support women to make autonomous and informed decisions irrespective of their own beliefs regarding the most appropriate method."*

It is not stated in what way the health professionals expected the women to be fully informed, nor why they believed that their professional opinion about a medical procedure constituted a "belief" as opposed to their professional knowledge. There is also the question of how the practitioners would determine the informed status of the woman if they didn't ask questions or advise.

A similar scenario is revealed by Martin;[94] a worker describes being involved in an abortion procedure where the woman was crying and upset. The worker says,

> *"///the doctor went to tell her, 'you don't have to do this, it can be fixed,' but that's not his job. His job is to do what she asked."*

---

93 Newton, Bayly, McNamee, Hardiman, Bismark, Webster, and Keogh, How do women seeking abortion choose.
94 Martin, Hassinger, Debbink and Harris, Dangertalk.

Some will reveal anonymously what they would never say publicly such as this outspoken regional abortion provider who admitted to me,

> *"Of course it's bad medicine, but if we are going to ensure it's available that's how we have to do it."*

There is a personal cost to the self-censorship involved in toeing the line. All the practitioners I interviewed for my research talked about their concerns for their clients in their interactions. However, some were also conscious of the toll it was taking on themselves to be so constantly on guard or feeling as though they had to compromise themselves in some way.

> *"I'm forced to live such an internal conflict because I believe the science that says there is no health benefit to this path for women, and potentially some serious harm. I can't tell her that, well I can, but I risk my career. How is that even good medicine?"*
> *(General Practitioner)*

The effects on people required to constantly self-censor on issues of such importance to them should not be underestimated. Bar Tal[95] cites a number of negative effects of self-censoring including an increase in personal distress when it is known that information is being withheld. Personal distress can also manifest as guilt and shame if the withheld information is considered to be significant.

Bar Tal also talks about the effects on society of the self-censorship of individuals in preventing the free flow of information, the decreasing of transparency, and the reinforcement of particular dogmas and ideologies. Self-censorship is both an outcome of Alarmist Gatekeeping and one of the most powerful mechanism for perpetuating the Dominant view.

95 Bar-Tal, Self-Censorship.

Practitioners experience a range of significant professional pressures to toe the line even in the absence of conscientious objection or legislation that compels an action. Practitioners often have to be registered with professional bodies which have policies or statements in support of abortion. Not all practitioners agree with the position and feel this means they would not be supported to do what they thought was the 'right thing' if they deemed this to be contrary to toeing the line.

> *"It was well known what the official position was at the uni when I was studying, and the AASW make it clear there's only one position we can take." (Social Worker)*

The professional body referred to here is the Australian Association of Social Workers which has a position statement on abortion declaring it a human right:

> *"Social work is founded on the principles of social justice, human rights and professional integrity. Women's access to reproductive health services, including abortion, cannot be separated from fundamental human rights and social justice. "*

The Australian Nursing and Midwifery Federation have also been firm Adherents to the Dominant Discoursing position and although they support the right of a nurse to conscientiously object to participation in abortion, they also actively support abortion rights, including the implementation of safe access zones and conscientious objection legislation.[96]

> *"There's not a hope the nurse's body would back me*

---

96 Australian Nursing and Midwifery Federation (SA Branch). (13 Nov 2020). ANMF Welcomes Safe Access Zone Laws. *ANMFSA* https://www.anmfsa.org.au/Web/News/2020/ANMF_welcomes_safe_access_zone_laws.aspx

up if I complained about that. They'd toe their own line, not support a nurse who suggested abortion isn't necessarily good for everyone. We all know it."
(Nurse)

While the strategies of Censoring and Discrediting are effective in maintaining the silence of those who threaten abortion rights, it is an uneasy silence that carries with it a personal cost that may have far-reaching consequences for those who self-censor.

"I wish I could change the past because things like this wreck a part of your soul, it leaves you with a sadness and regret that you can't explain to anyone who hasn't done this." (Anne)

Walking the Tightrope

It is the subtle, the covert, the unwritten rules, the things that "I can't quite put my finger on," things that "aren't quite right" that may hold the most power in terms of encouraging a process of internalised censorship. This is undoubtedly true for the individual practitioners who sometimes found it difficult to articulate precisely what their concerns were, or why they interacted with clients in specific ways.

> *"I'm usually conscious of not putting anyone off with my response or making them think that I'm going to... that I sit on one particular side of the fence... that can be alienating, so yep, there are some things I don't say that... maybe now that I think about it... maybe should be said... but I don't say them because well... I guess they might not hear them the way I intend?"*

The ways in which practitioners balance their responsibilities to clients and the perceived risk to themselves or to abortion rights has been described as like "walking a tightrope" and what this may mean for women who are seeking information or support is significant. Such internalised censorship means that women have few sources of information about the potential of adverse impacts on their physical or mental health or their relationships. Because of the Alarmist Gatekeeping strategy of Discrediting information about adverse effects of abortion, women may also view with suspicion any information about risk, no matter how accurate.

Management of perception was very important to the majority of practitioners and generally resulted in interactions that ensured compliance or toeing the line by avoiding specific topics or withholding certain information. Some practitioners were clear that some subjects were more off-limits than others.

> *"Well, foetal development is one thing that I actually think is important to many women, but now I often don't bring it up. It's one of those things people think are 'pro-lifey.'"(Nurse)*

> *"Yes, foetal development can be tricky. I wouldn't raise it on a phone call. I need to see the woman, see if she is comfortable with me and see her reactions to the information." (Social Worker)*

> *"Even if I suspect her emotional issues might be about the abortion, I wouldn't raise that if I thought she was too vulnerable. All it takes is one of the other workers to hear that, and there would probably be a complaint, and the client would feel like I'd betrayed her if she was told differently by someone else." (Mental Health Nurse)*

Concern about perception was not limited to what the woman might think, but how the woman might interpret or misinterpret the interaction or how others that she talks to might do the same. When listening to the concerns of practitioners about what they say, to whom they say it, and who might discover it, it is easy to see the concept of Foucault's panopticism at work. In Bentham's work on his vision of the panopticon, an integral aspect was that power should be "visible and unverifiable," leaving one aware that the power exists, but never sure when or where it will be wielded.

> *"I worry as much about the fact that the people she talks to after she talks to me understand what I've said as I do that she understands what I'm saying." (General Practitioner)*

> *"There's also the problem of her going off and seeing someone else in the future and saying, "Well, J said that I wasn't properly informed, or properly screened" or something similar... and that person telling her that the reason she suffered is because of what I said... not because of what happened." (Counsellor)*

In the setting of a number of pregnancy centres being targeted by a Queensland MP, as previously discussed, one practitioner says,

> *"I'm second guessing everything I do now. I'm finding it more difficult to connect with clients because I'm always asking myself if this is a setup and to be very careful. It's not that I've ever said, or been accused of saying anything wrong... it's just that, if I say this, can they twist it to sound like something else?" (Social Worker)*

While all of the practitioners stated that they would never engage in manipulative behaviours, many commented that it was the appearance of being manipulative that was important.

> *"I'm very conscious of not being persuasive or pushing."*

> *"I don't want to appear manipulative."*

> *"It is really really important that we don't appear manipulative."*

> *"If a woman was asking me what I thought I would say that to make the decision that's best for you its best for you to talk to someone about it... but I would never say... 100% I would never say I've seen women suffering after it, that would be manipulative."*

"Manipulative" in this case was determined in some cases by whether they engaged in informing women even when the decision not to mention a possible risk factor potentially compromised the practitioner's informed consent responsibility:

> *"I wouldn't tell a woman that she may suffer negative effects necessarily... because I may set her up for that... yes, even though I know it's a possibility... if she was saying "this is what I'm doing" [have an abortion] and didn't seem interested in more information, I wouldn't say anything, especially if her values seemed more aligned with abortion."*

One practitioner said that he refuses to take referrals of women considering abortion after finding himself "floundering about what was okay to say" with such clients previously. Another practitioner said that when asked about their reproductive histories, clients could be very tearful if disclosing an abortion. She talked about this being so common that it was concerning. She also expressed confidence that she was sure other more experienced practitioners would provide appropriate support, stating that she believed abortion providers to be the best source of information for women.

All practitioners were able to recall having seen clients who had disclosed an abortion experience at some point, and each was conscious of having had a heightened sense of awareness about it which made them more conscious about what they said and how they said it. For one social worker, abortion took on a very different ambience in the interaction, describing it as "a shade darker than everything else," and "it's always in the room, even if we don't address it directly."

For another practitioner, it was the incongruency she saw in some of the women that was significant:

> *"I just watched the tears pouring out of her, and he [the partner] was oblivious. I didn't know how to point it out when she was clearly saying words that made it okay, but the pain was leaching out of her."(Counsellor/Nurse)*

Most practitioners experienced a sense of helplessness about how to help a woman in these circumstances, at the same time knowing that few other people would be equipped to support her either:

> *"In many ways, it's sadder to see these patients because everyone has given up on them… to help them before they get here. And they're nearly all convinced they deserve to be in so much pain because they made the choice." (General Practitioner)*

> *"There's no question that the woman is suffering, but the system doesn't allow any way for that feedback so that suffering can be known." (Counsellor)*

It is important to understand that while so many practitioners censor anything they or others may percieve as threatening to the Principle, many women experience extremes of coercion like Joelle...

> *"I was told AT my 12 week screen that I needed to proceed with further testing quickly in order to 'make decisions' about our pregnancy.*
>
> *The seed was planted THERE.*
>
> ***I was given NO hope*** *that my baby would survive at 13 weeks. I was told she was in heart failure and full of fluid, and said it would be best to end the pregnancy.*
>
> *At 14 weeks, after a confirmed diagnosis of Down syndrome, I was encouraged to delay my travel plans back to Queensland so that an abortion within 48 hours could be enacted.*
>
> ***When I said no, the pressure stepped up.***
>
> *At 14.5 weeks the doctor said 'I don't know why the receptionist even gave you a blue book' (the medical book every pregnant woman received to track their pregnancy). I was again told there was no hope and that it would be best to end her life.*
>
> *Then I was informed of how to make sure I collected all parts of my baby to take in to hospital when I miscarried. At 15 weeks I was checked on again by the hospital via phone. I was told that what I was doing (by not choosing abortion) was keeping her until 'foetal demise' occurred. Basically she wouldn't develop and would pass naturally.*

At 19 weeks when she looked like her heart was ok and the excess fluid situation had resolved, I imagined I wouldn't receive any more coercion about abortion from medical professionals.

I was wrong. At every weekly appointment from 19 weeks to 23 weeks I was asked if I was sure I wanted to proceed with her pregnancy. was even told that 'these things happen' in second marriages and asked if her father and I were a second marriage.

Not once were we given information about Down syndrome, not once. Despite resources available from our state Down syndrome organisation that could have helped, I wasn't even told about organisations, let along current information.

Despite me pleading for information, I was told to go home and google her diagnosis. At her birth the same doctor that asked if I was in a second marriage entered the birthing suite as the delivery doctor.

Once Josee was born she was smitten. Every time we saw her after she was intrigued by Josec Hope… Why? Because the obstetricians that we encountered didn't have a lived experience of the condition.

Why do I spend SO much of my time trying to convey the inadequacies of prenatal information, care and support when it comes to babies with Down syndrome? Because I endured so much negative stigma, out dated perceptions and coercion in my pregnancy.

I could have ended her life easily because abortion was offered at EVERY turn, and because I was made to feel like it was the right thing to do...by the same professionals that should have been objectively informing me and providing optimal prenatal clinical care.

Think of the most frustrating situation you've ever been in.

Now imagine that when you try and speak up about it people shut you down and say you have no right to judge.

That's how I feel every time I advocate.

WAKE up Australia and realise the level of coercion taking place in pregnancies right now." (Joelle)

Sadly such coercion toward abortion is very common and while Adherents advocate abortion for babies like Josee Hope, the messages we send people living full lives with these conditions is shocking.

Conscientious Objection

Alarmist Gatekeeping can lead to legislative acts that serve the Dominant Discourse, often perpetuating the negative consequences. In the case of abortion, legislation has significantly silenced many who might raise genuine concerns, or who could provide scientific information, emotional or material support, alternative options, or just a listening ear. Such legislative Acts further reinforce the notion that dissenters from the Dominant Discourse are wrong, and in fact so wrong that they may be subject to criminal proceedings. This is a very powerful censorship tool with very serious consequences to women.

Some practitioners felt it had become considered manipulative even to ask a woman if she had considered not having an abortion.

> *"I used to say 'congratulations' to my patients. Now I have to say, 'What would you like to do?' It's all wrong." (General Practitioner)*

> *"I don't see a lot of good modelling for young women... that there is a support system and motherhood can be positive even when it's hard. Who's even allowed to tell them that anymore?" (Counsellor/ Nurse)*

Some deal directly with the legal requirements imposed on them by conscientious objection laws by informing clients and allowing them to decide what they want to hear:

> *"I've found a way to be able to tell a patient that the law tells me I'm supposed to refer her even if I think it may be risky. She invariably asks me what I mean. Mostly I have good relationships with them, and I'm able to explain the evidence of harm and feel relatively confident they understand my position. Not always, but mostly. It isn't without risks though."*
> *(General Practitioner)*

Conscientious Objection is defined by the Australian Medical Association as a position based on "sincerely held beliefs and moral concerns" that "conflict with their peer-based professional practice." Such "sincerely held beliefs" have been the subject of legislative action ostensibly to protect women's access to abortion from doctors who are perceived to impede such access, regardless of their actual reasons for concern.

The Victorian Abortion Law Reform Act of 2008 states the following:

(1)   If a woman requests a registered health practitioner to advise on a proposed abortion, or to perform, direct, authorise or supervise an abortion for that woman, and the practitioner has a conscientious objection to abortion, the practitioner must:

    (a)   Inform the woman that the practitioner has a conscientious objection to abortion, and:

    (b)   Refer the woman to another registered health practitioner in the same regulated health profession who the practitioner knows does not have a conscientious objection to abortion.

The inference of this legislation is not only that the unwillingness to refer for abortion is innately harmful, regardless of the reason, but that a health practitioner who does not ultimately refer, cannot even advise a woman on abortion.

The Australian Medical Association[97] reinforced this when they advised Victorian doctors after the enactment of these laws that:

> *"If it becomes clear that a patient you are seeing is wanting help with a termination, you must stop the consultation at that point and advise you have a conflict."*

It is then further asserted that an alternate doctor who has no conscientious objection to abortion is better able to assess the woman's needs:

> *"Doctors who are troubled by this should remember that at the Family Planning clinic the patient will be discussing her pregnancy with another doctor, and regardless of her intentions from the outset, it is not a certainty that she will proceed with a termination. If you refer her as soon as you become aware she may be considering a termination, (that is, if you refrain from any further discussion) you are in fact referring her to Family Planning for advice on her pregnancy."*

This has the effect of reinforcing the perspective that a doctor who holds a belief against abortion or a concern about a specific

---

97 Australian Medical Association (2013). Conscientious Objection Policy 15. Cited in White, C., Stewart, C. and Diamond, S. K. (19 Aug 2013). Reproductive Health (Access to Terminations) Inquiry [Transcript]. Committee Room 2, Parliament House, Hobart. p14. https://www.parliament.tas.gov.au/ctee/council/Transcripts/19%20August%20 2013%20-%20Hobart1.pdf

patient with regard to abortion, even a concern based on sound medical evidence, cannot be trusted to provide a woman with accurate information about the procedure or her options. One Expert suggests that values should not be employed in one's professional decision making at all:

> *"Values are important parts of our lives. But values and conscience have different roles in public and private life. They should influence discussion on what kind of health system to deliver. But they should not influence the care an individual doctor offers to his or her patient. The door to value-driven medicine is a door to a Pandora's box of idiosyncratic, bigoted, discriminatory medicine."*[98]

He goes on to say that, *"Public servants [meaning doctors] must act in the public interest, not their own."* Of course, this statement, along with legislation to silence people who hold specified values, is underpinned by its own values, something the author fails to acknowledge. Many doctors can have concerns about their patients seeking abortion for a variety of reasons specific to that patient, without such concern being based on 'values.'

Regardless of the provided definition, there is ambiguity in what constitutes an objection to abortion, including issues of overlap between a health practitioner's possible moral concerns about abortion and a known patient's risk factors for abortion. Even in the absence of moral concerns about abortion, if a health practitioner holds concerns about a patient's personal risk factors or coercive factors in her life, that doctor may still perceive a legal duty to refer on.

In effect, this means that any woman enquiring about abortion, whether she has made up her mind, or is seeking counsel, or

---

98 Savulescu, J. (2006). Conscientious Objection in Medicine, *BMJ*, 332:294.

really wanting support to carry the baby to term, is by law put on a path directly to an abortion provider.

> *"Once I've seen her if she even gets to see me, she moves down that conveyor belt fairly quickly, things are arranged very quickly, not a lot of thinking time. Like the woman has almost no part of it… it happens to her." (Mental Health Nurse)*

When laws exist that state that a doctor who does not agree with abortion, whether for religious, ethical, or medical reasons, cannot be trusted to provide accurate information about abortion, abortion discourse becomes the sole domain of those more concerned with 'rights' than with women themselves.

One of the more significant issues in legislation of this kind is the question of at what point any health professional is able to say "no" to a woman requesting an abortion, even when it is deemed risky to her physical or mental health. While ostensibly a law for conscientious objectors it will also be a law that could create fear in any doctor with legitimate concerns for their patient.

We see that such concerns are valid when Adherents begin suggesting that conscientious objection is simply an excuse to opt out of abortion referral. Abortion providers in one study criticised the use of conscientious objection as a *"convenient excuse"* to opt out of abortion service provision and stated that there need to be limits on conscientious objection.[99] There is no acknowledgement of valid reasons that doctors may have for not recommending or referring for abortion, nor of any impingement on the right of the doctor to their professional perspective.

There was, however, acknowledgment from one participant that even without a practitioner referral on to an abortion provider

---

99 Keogh, L., Gillam, L., Bismark, M., McNamee, K., Webster, A., Bayly, C. & Newton, D. (2019). Conscientious Objection to Abortion, the Law and its Implementation in Victoria, Australia: Perspectives of Abortion Service Providers. *Medical Ethics*, 20:11.

there is nothing to stop the woman from finding out information for herself, "because it is pretty easy to find out if you just turn on your computer."[100]

One practitioner who had worked with many women struggling to cope after an abortion experience questioned whose responsibility it is supposed to be to tell a woman that it doesn't always turn out as she expected:

> *"The doctors should not only know this information; they should be giving it... but we know they're not... and we can't trust them to do it... so how are they ever expected to know?" (Social Worker)*

With abortion often referred to as a decision between a woman and her doctor, there is a considerable inconsistency when professional bodies advise doctors to avoid even talking to their patient but to refer them on immediately. This means that it is possible that there may be no point at which risk factors for adverse psychological harm for a woman are assessed or that she is informed of these. There are many examples in the Discourse where doctors abrogate their responsibility to inform or assess women attending for abortion, including from women who say they only saw the doctor:

> *"... after sitting for hours in a waiting room, then all he did was hand me the bloody pill. I don't even remember him saying anything to me. It was like I wasn't even there. "(Simone)*

There is also a failure to ensure that she has access to information about all available alternatives including community organisations that may be able to meet some of the needs driving her

---

100 Keogh, Gillam, Bismark, McNamee, Webster, Bayly, and Newton, Conscientious Objection to Abortion.

toward abortion if they are social or economic. Many such services are available free of charge through pregnancy support organisations which are actively Discredited by Adherents.

Information about risk factors, whether evidence-based or not, is often labelled paternalistic by Adherents. It is common for those who provide such information to be accused of manipulative and misleading behaviours. We see this in the example of research linking abortion with adverse psychological harm. The veracity of such information is irrelevant. It would seem misleading to advise women there is no evidence of a risk factor when in fact such evidence does exist.

A number of Australian professional bodies deny such links, while at the same time listing risk factors for the potential of harm, which itself is inconsistent. A recommendation from the Queensland Government[101] that women should be followed up post-abortively, subsequent to reported suicides of women after abortion, is also inconsistent with denials of the evidence of harm.

> *"... women who are at risk of mental health problems may fall through the gaps between termination providers..."*

> *"... explore how communication between (other health services and) termination of pregnancy providers could be enhanced to ensure women are appropriately supported after a termination of pregnancy."*

In their discussion paper on pregnancy termination, the Royal Australian and New Zealand College of Psychiatrists (RANZCP)

---

101 Humphrey, M., Colditz, P., Flenady, V. and Whelan, N. (2013). *Maternal and Perinatal Mortality and Morbidity in Queensland: Queensland Maternal and Perinatal Quality Council Report 2013*. Department of Health, State of Queensland.

acknowledges that there are a "number of well-respected studies that have found definite psychiatric sequelae" and suggest that consideration should be given to a woman's particular risk factors when seeking an abortion.[102] The RANZCP also contributed a submission to the Queensland Government in favour of decriminalisation of abortion but suggesting pre- and post-counselling support. One authority often referred to by Australian Adherents is the American Psychological Association which denies harmful psychological effects to the average woman having a first-trimester abortion, and then lists risk factors for harmful psychological effects.[103]

This adds to the confusion for some practitioners:

> *"So, how do I assess a woman's risk factors if there is no evidence she might have issues anyway? Do they even hear what they are saying?" (General Practitioner)*

Another practitioner described other issues such as vaccination or circumcision or breastfeeding versus bottle feeding as potentially sensitive for a client, but "nothing like abortion" and there wasn't the same sense of having to "walk a tightrope" in the discussions.

> *"I don't even think about whether it's okay to share my professional opinion on any other issue. It's my job." (General Practitioner)*

In spite of the evidence of potential harm from abortion, there is no acknowledgement that there exist women who may be better

---

102 The Royal Australian and New Zealand College of Psychiatrists (March 2011*). Discussion Paper: Termination of Pregnancy.* https://www.ranzcp.org/files/resources/reports/termination_of_pregnancy-pdf.aspx

103 American Psychological Association (2008). *APA Task Force Finds Single Abortion Not a Threat to Women's Mental Health.* https://www.apa.org/news/press/releases/2008/08/single-abortion

served by practitioners who, in their professional capacity, determine that not all women are best served by accessing abortion, whether because they are being coerced or because they have a psychosocial need that could be better met.

"Knowing what I know now, it's a decision that I took too lightly and made too easily. There should be someone who makes sure you know EXACTLY what you are doing and you should be made to speak to women who have done it.

I wish I could change the past because things like this wreck a part of your soul, it leaves you with a sadness and regret that you can't explain to anyone who hasn't done this." (Lauren)

Legislating Censorship
and Dissent

As can be seen with conscientious objection laws, some of the more concerning consequences of Alarmist Gatekeeping are seen in the power of the Dominant view to influence legislative change. Over the past decade, laws have been enacted in a number of states making it illegal to talk about abortion within certain distances of an abortion clinic and compelling doctors to make abortion referrals. The legislative change discussed here have been a result of both the deception of Adherents and a disturbing censorship of information placed before or accepted by legislators. None of these laws have any evidence of benefit for women, and I argue that in fact they impinge on the rights of many women and others in the community.

The drive for legislative change on the issue of abortion is generally based on the principle of rights and perceived autonomy of women. Yet such rights and autonomy are not legislated for in other aspects of reproductive health practice. It is accepted for doctors to refuse specific interventions when they believe that either the risks are higher than the benefits, or when they simply believe a woman may change her mind.

In the case of tubal ligation (female sterilisations), for example,

O'Connor[104] states that the common practice among practitioners is to refuse the procedure to women under the age of 30. The article in which this appeared is a publication produced by RANZCOG and a major abortion advocacy organisation. It was brought to my attention by one of the practitioners I interviewed.

> *"So this article, 'The importance of saying no,' sends me the message about how important it is to make sure my patients validly consent and are informed of all risks… on every other issue, but not abortion? How am I supposed to carry out my duty of care if the AMA says I should refer straight away? How do I make sure any other doctor knows about my patient's risks? I know they won't even ask her. Who is responsible for that?" (General Practitioner)*

Decriminalisation of abortion has been based on Disinformation claiming that women have limited access and are suffering stigma in abortion access due to its inclusion in the Criminal Code. Commentary on the issue in social media (detailed later in this chapter) demonstrates that this is not the reality of experience for most women. However, the greater normalisation of abortion which occurs through legal sanctions can have a more sinister impact:

> *"I felt no pressure toward abortion, except by virtue of the fact that it seemed so "normal," so available. At the time I was a little annoyed that I'd had to travel to Melbourne for it (two hours away), but it was only a minor inconvenience. Now I see so many things differently. I am only just beginning to understand that* what I did was betray my unborn child,

104 O'Connor, M. (2016). The Importance of Saying No. *O&G Magazine*, The Royal Australian and New Zealand College of Obstetricians and Gynaecologists, 18(3):16-18.

*potentially the little girl I'd sometimes wished for.
I'm a little numb about it right now. I'm not really
sure where to go to talk about it. I think about all the
times one young client of mine used to want to cry to
me about her "baby" and I would tell her about the
"choice" she made and that it was valid and okay...
I denied her her grief, just as right now I am not
able to face my own." (Felicity)*

For women like Felicity there is a very subtle coercion at play. Abortion is simple to get with just a phone call, whether decriminalised or not. However, in Victoria, where she accessed her abortion, the way in which any activity which doesn't actively promote abortion has been criminalised also had an impact. She went on to say,

*"I learned to filter out anything negative about
abortion early on in my work with women and this
was helped when the laws changed as well. If it was
illegal to tell women negative things about abortion, then surely it had to all be completely false.
Now I wonder how much of that is actually true."*

There are currently specific references to legal restriction regarding abortion in all states and territories of Australia. An exception is the Australian Capital Territory where the only mention is in regard to the qualification of those performing abortions, and facilities where they can be undertaken.[105] Every other state and territory has guidelines or restrictions on gestational limits, while essentially decriminalising abortion within those restrictions. New South Wales is the only state where abortion remainswithin the Criminal Code.[106] This Act does not specify when an abortion

105 Australian Capital Territory (2002). Medical Practitioners (Maternal Health) Amendment Bill 2002.
106   New South Wales Government (1900). New South Wales Crimes Act. https://

might be considered lawful, however case law based on a decision in 1971 by Justice Levine, known as the Levine ruling, means it is generally accepted that abortion was.

> *"//not unlawful if a doctor honestly believed on reasonable grounds that "the operation was necessary to preserve the woman involved from serious danger to her life or physical or mental health which the continuance of pregnancy would entail."[107]*

"Mental health" has since been interpreted to include "the effects of economic or social stress that may pertain either during pregnancy or after birth."[108] Abortion is lawful if performed to prevent *"serious danger to the woman's mental and physical health"* which includes economic and social pressures. Similar interpretations operated in other states prior to decriminalisation. In practice the legal threshold is so low that the law makes no difference and many women are unaware there are any legal restrictions at all, as demonstrated below.

In Australia, legislative change comes about for a variety of reasons. The Australian Law Reform Commission identifies three primary motivators for the reform, development, or updating of laws:[109]

1. Community concern about a particular issue that needs to be addressed through the process of law reform;
2. Events or legal cases which highlight a deficiency in the law;
3. Scientific or technological developments that make new laws necessary.

---

www.legislation.nsw.gov.au/view/html/inforce/current/act-1900-040
107 R v Wald [1971]
108 CES v Superclinics Australia Pty. Ltd [1995]. http://www8.austlii.edu.au/cgi-bin/viewdoc/au/cases/nsw/NSWSC/1995/103.html
109 Australian Law Reform Commission (2020). *Law Reform Process*. https://www.alrc.gov.au/about/law-reform-process/

Abortion law in Australia is governed by state governments, all of which have their own version of Law Reform Commissions. However, the principles for legislative change remain the same. Adherent moves for legislative reform are generally based on the first two points above, with statements that abortion law is "out of step with community attitudes" and that access will be improved if the law changes.

> *"... the process is unnecessarily scary, complex and stigmatised, and only occurs at all because of a tenuous legal loophole."[110]*

> *"... it [criminalisation of abortion] puts women's health and lives at risk, especially if they live in rural and remote areas where timely terminations are notoriously hard to access."[111]*

> *"Surely a law that is so widely and routinely disobeyed is—by any definition—an ineffective law and completely out of step with reality."[112]*

This last statement is particularly disturbing, given that it clearly articulates that many abortions are slipping through current systems and being undertaken illegally. Abortion providers are obviously demonstrating little regard for legislation at any point.

In 2008 abortion was decriminalised in the State of Victoria, making abortion available to 24 weeks for any reason, and after 24 weeks with the agreement of two doctors.[113] It was anticipated that decriminalisation would, among other things, make abortion more accessible to women and decrease the stigma surrounding

---

110 Bannister, L. (2 Jun 2017). Australian Lawmakers Vote No on Legal Abortion Law, *Teen Vogue*.

111 Caro, Two Heated Issues Down.

112 Caro, Two Heated Issues Down.

113 Victorian Government (2008). Abortion Law Reform Act 2008. http://www5.austlii.edu.au/au/legis/vic/consol_act/alra2008209/

the procedure.[114]

It was evident four years later that decriminalisation had failed to achieve these goals and, in fact, some believed that service provision had decreased:

> *"Since abortion law reform access to public services has shrunk. It's not getting better. It's shrunk."[115]*

In 2012, Expert Leslie Cannold who spearheaded a number of campaigns to decriminalise abortion as the head of a reproductive rights organisation wrote:[116] "I'*m no longer convinced that changing the law is enough to destroy the stigma and shaming that surrounds abortion.*" Based on the fact that little has changed on the [abortion] service provision front, she goes on to state that, "*indeed, it may be that criminal sanctions on abortion don't cause abortion shaming and stigma.*"

In spite of this reality, the lead-up to decriminalisation in Queensland was met with the same strategies of Alarmism, Disinformation, and Misinformation that dominated the Discourse in other states, with Adherent organisations and individuals calling for law reform as a solution to both access and stigma.

> *"Women… could not access a safe procedure."[117]*

114 Keogh, L., Newton, D., Bayly, C., McNamee, K., Hardiman, A., Webster, A. and Bismark, M. (2017). Intended and Unintended Consequences of Abortion Law Reform: Perspectives of Abortion Experts in Victoria, Australia. *Journal of Family Planning and Reproductive Health Care*; 43(18):18-24.

115 Keogh, Newton, Bayly, McNamee, Hardiman, Webster, and Bismark, Intended and Unintended Consequences.

116 Cannold, L. (18 Sept 2012). Abortion Shaming, What the Law Does and Doesn't Do. *Right Now.* http://rightnow.org.au/opinion-3/abortion-shaming-what-the-law-does-and-doesn%e2%80%99t-do/#disqus_thread

117 Children by Choice (2016). *Submission to the Health, Communities, Disability Services and Domestic and Family Violence Prevention Committee, Review of Termination of Pregnancy Laws.* https://docplayer.net/25527962-Abortion-law-reform-women-s-right-to-choose-amendment-bill-2016.html

> *"..stigma is still attached to abortion, which contin-*
> *ued criminality helps perpetuate."[118]*

> *"Removal of terminations from the criminal code*
> *will "provide more timely access to treatment*
> *options and decrease the need for travel."[119]*

When the information being used to support legislative change
is so inconsistent and used in such misleading ways, we must
always question whether other agendas are at play.

118 Children by Choice (2016). *Submission to the Health, Communities, Disability Services and Domestic and Family Violence Prevention Committee, Review of Termination
of Pregnancy Laws.* https://docplayer.net/25527962-Abortion-law-reform-women-s-
right-to-choose-amendment-bill-2016.html
119 Marie Stopes (2018). Submission to the Health, Communities, Disability Services
and Domestic and Family Violence Prevention Committee, Review of Termination of
Pregnancy Laws.

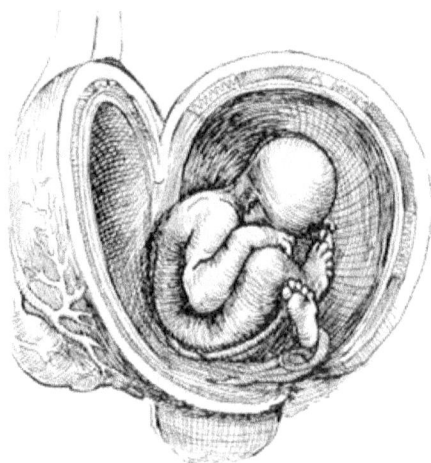

"Technically Illegal"

In order to advocate for decriminalisation in any state where the process has been undertaken or attempted, Adherents generally use alarmist and misleading information to sway both the public and politicians.

> *"By restricting safe, legal options, women's lives are literally endangered."[120]*

> *"... it [abortion being in the Criminal Code] puts women's health and lives at risk."[121]*

> *"No woman should ever be put in a position whereby she is forced to go through a pregnancy she does not want or risk her own life to stop it."[122]*

The assertions that medical practitioners or women fear reprisals or are too scared to access services is contradicted by the many messages women themselves give, particularly in social media in response to such articles. The following comments were provided on a public Facebook page to a woman seeking information about accessing abortion in Queensland prior to decriminalisation:[123]

120 Noyes, The Women of NSW Deserve Better.
121 Caro, Two Heated Issues Down.
122 Noyes, The Women of NSW Deserve Better.
123   Imperfect Mums Facebook group. n.d.

> *"There are Marie Stopes clinics that advertise them on their website. Not illegal at all!"*

> *"It's technically illegal, but they are straight forward to get, no referral needed for private clinics."*

> *"No they aren't. They are perfectly legal in QLD not sure where you got your information from."*

> *"They are not illegal."*

> *"You can walk into ANY clinic in Queensland that performs this procedure with an appointment and have the procedure done."*

> *"Yes, it's "technically illegal" however, you do not need a referral, you will not be arrested, you will not be charged with a crime."*

> *"Yeah, no they're completely legal in QLD."*

The quotes above are only a few of more than 100 comments on one post where a woman had asked for advice about an unintended pregnancy. This selection reflects the majority of comments which demonstrate the clear understanding that whether legal or not, abortion is easy to access and not stigmatised as criminal.

The parliamentary speeches by Queensland Ministers of Parliament in support of decriminalisation were replete with misinformation. Two MPs misrepresented information provided by a Victorian MP:

> *"As abortion is a legal procedure, the Victorian government has been able to accurately capture statistics on the number of women accessing terminations.*

> *In Victoria, the 10-year trend shows that legalising abortion reduces the rate of abortion. The statistics show a reduction from 16.8 procedures per 1000 women in 2008 to 12.2 procedures in 2017. The evidence is clear."[124]*

The letter from which they derived this information cautioned that the Victorian government censors statistical information because of "the sensitive nature of the issues involved" and "the limitations of the datasets." The letter further cautions that if the contained information which suggests a reduction in abortion statistics is published, the limitations must also be stated. One of these limitations refers to the fact that only surgical abortions are reflected in the figures between 2008 and 2017. With significant increases in medical abortion in that decade, the suggestion that there has been an overall decrease in abortion is guesswork at best. Using this as a reason to promote decriminalisation is clearly misinformed.

Queensland MP Jackie Trad who put forward the Bill for decriminalisation labelled the speech of one Senator opposing the Bill as "hate speech." The transcript of this speech in its entirety is reproduced here for the importance of understanding such labelling by Adherents.

> *"Thank you one and all for being here to send a clear message to all those who govern, that children matter. We know that the measure of a society is how we treat those who cannot speak for themselves. Now that includes some people who are ill or disabled. It includes the aged. It includes children, but it must also include the unborn. In so many*

---

124 Pugh, J. (2018). *Daily Hansard.* https://www.parliament.qld.gov.au/documents/hansard/2018/2018_10_16_WEEKLY.pdf

ways, we as a society have dropped the ball on this important measure. Elder abuse is rising. Children in care face enormous life challenges, and we particularly failed Aboriginal children living in some of Australia's remote communities.

Children and babies may not be able to vote, but we must ensure that they are heard and protected by all those who govern. A grown man or woman is capable of the agency required to make decisions about their sexual conduct, contraception, and the consequences thereof, but a child who is the product of those decisions has no such agency. And it is incumbent upon those who speak, who can speak, to defend their interests always. I'm so grateful that all of you are here to speak and to show how much we support those who cannot speak for themselves.

We know the most fundamental human right is the right to life itself. Article 6 of the International Covenant on Civil and Political Rights provides that every human being has the inherent right to life. This right shall be protected by law.

No one shall be arbitrarily deprived of his life. This is our most basic responsibility at international law. It's meant to underpin all of the laws of this land. So attempts in this context to suggest that a foetus is something less than human, are a mere justification, flying in the face of the scientific investment and progress that has been made to ensure the viability of prematurely born babies.

The focus of lawmakers in Queensland should be on how women facing unplanned pregnancy can be supported into making decisions to either raise a child or to offer a child for adoption to the very many couples we know who face infertility.

I promised to be brief, so I shall finish where I began. The measure of our society is what we do to speak for, to protect those who cannot speak for themselves. Thank you so much for being here to fight for it today. Thank you."[125]

It would be challenging for most thinking people to identify this as "hate speech" unless their agenda is purely one of denigrating the speaker. The same Adherent MP has in more recent times labelled a Queensland pro-life organisation, Cherish Life, as a "vicious organisation" on her Facebook page. The agenda of those who promote abortions become clearer when such Discrediting is exposed, particularly when the target is someone who is either providing factual evidence, expressing concerns reflective of many in the community or even proposing that women require more support.

Many of the submissions received in support of decriminalisation lament the stigma, limited access, prohibitive cost, and geographic disparity in abortion access for many women as though the law at the time was responsible for these issues. They frequently referred to the need to make the legislative change in order to increase access and better support women, even though there is no evidence that either of these results has occurred in the setting of decriminalisation in other states. Not only was the process replete with misinformation and alarmism, but there were also conscious and strategic steps taken to censor specific

---

125 Stoker, A. (March 2018). Speech given at Queensland pro-life rally.

information.

The Health Committee tasked with gathering information to inform parliament before the Queensland decriminalisation vote had made it clear before receiving any submissions that they were approaching the process from a censorious position. In the lead-up to decriminalisation of abortion in Queensland, the Health Committee request for submissions stated:

> *"The committee has resolved not to accept images of foetuses or the outcomes of medical procedures."*[126]

While the statement is that such images or information would not be accepted, a number of submissions containing these were submitted and subsequently censored before being published on the website. The censorship of submissions, however, went a lot further than blacking out foetal images. It extended to the removal of words, facts about medical and surgical procedures, and even links to published studies.

The World Federation of Doctors Who Respect Human Life made a submission to the Queensland Health Committee arguing against the proposed decriminalisation Bill (Submission No. 461). The submission was provided on their organisational letterhead that contains a well-known Da Vinci drawing of an unborn baby.

Not only was the image itself blacked out of the published submission, but even the words which described it, "foetus in the womb," were censored. Within the 18-page submission, more than two dozen sections were blacked out, including accurate medical descriptions and names of abortion procedures, direct quotes from abortion providers describing procedures, names of

---

126 Queensland Parliament (2018). *Report No. 11, 56ᵗʰ Parliament – Termination of Pregnancy Bill 2018. Inquiry Overview.* https://www.parliament.qld.gov.au/work-of-committees/committees/HCDSDFVPC/inquiries/past-inquiries/TerminationOfPregnancyB18

television shows that were referred to, referenced journal articles, and one post-abortive woman's experience of waking up after an abortion.

The same Health Committee that saw fit to refuse to read, see, or hear information that did not fit the Dominant agenda reported its findings back to parliament:[127]

> *"The current state of the law has created uncertainty among doctors and that the possibility of prosecution of health professionals and women potentially impedes provision of a full range of safe, accessible and timely reproductive services."*

> *"… the lack of certainty under the current provisions as to when a termination is lawful negatively impacts the accessibility and availability of termination services by causing fear and stigma for women, and reluctance by some health practitioners to provide such services."*

Abortion was subsequently decriminalised in yet another state. Whether one believes abortion should be in the Criminal Code or not, serious questions should be asked about the processes involved in the censorship of information and the perpetuation of misinformation that drives such change. When legislators only consider half the picture—the half that supports the proposed change—the public can never feel confident that their best interests are being served.

---

127 State of Queensland (2018). *Termination of Pregnancy Bill 2018, Explanatory Notes.* https://www.parliament.qld.gov.au/Documents/TableOffice/TabledPapers/2018/5618T1161.pdf

Safety or Censorship?

"When I stepped out of the taxi, I was gently approached by an older lady who handed me a brochure. Her only words were, "Do you really want to do this?" I burst into tears and said "No!" If not for the pro-life advocates outside that abortion clinic that day and the advice they offered about other options, I would also have ended that pregnancy—and my beautiful daughter would not be here today." (Nancy)

Media representations of those who congregate outside abortion clinics are an example of misinformation and Out-Grouping of Dissidents. While there is indeed evidence that some individuals carry out activities of a protest nature, the majority of known groups who undertake abortion clinic activity state that they are there to simply offer support to women. Other groups and individuals carry out a peaceful prayer vigil for what they deem to be the loss of lives of the unborn. A number of women like Nancy above have also come forward at different times with stories of having changed their mind about abortion, to continue a pregnancy as a result of such support.

Mainstream media reporting of activities outside abortion clinics label them in negative terms such as anti-abortion pro-testers or picketers, and accuse groups of abuse and harassment that harms or threatens women. This representation of all people outside abortion clinics, based on the actions of the occasional individual who may act in ways deemed inappropriate, have led to some states legislating to create what are termed "safe access zones." These are areas delineated by the distance from an abor-tion clinic within which it is illegal to carry out activities that have been determined as constituting a threat to women entering the clinic.

Such activity has been legislated not only in Victoria and Tasmania but also the Northern Territory, New South Wales, Queensland, and South Australia. Legislation limiting activities within a certain distance of abortion clinics are referred to in dif-ferent states as follows:

- Victoria: Public Health and Wellbeing Amendment (Safe Access Zones) Act 2015
- Tasmania: Reproductive Health (Access to Terminations) Act 2013
- New South Wales: Safe Access to Reproductive Health Clin-ics 2018
- Northern Territory: Safe Access Zones 2017
- ACT: Health (Patient Privacy) Amendment Bill
- Queensland: Safe Access Zones 2018
- South Australia: Safe Access Zones 2020

The terminology in using the words "safe access" in these Bills is Alarmist in itself, adding to the Discrediting messages about peo-ple outside clinics. The lack of evidence that women are harmed by people outside clinics reveals that they are hardly in need of "safety."

When two female Members of Parliament voted against the legislation of Safe Access Zones, the strategies of Alarmism and Out-Grouping were vociferous. These MPs were accused of having *"dodgy morals"* and of wanting women to be *"bullied and hounded."*[128]

> *"She's supposed to protect women and fight for their rights. But instead, Tanya Davies voted in favour of bullying and harassment."*[129]

> *"Two women, whose job it is to advocate for women and act in their best interests, actively tried to ensure NSW woman continued to be bullied and hounded."*[130]

> *"The decision of one of the MPs was described as "Un-f**cking believable" followed by the comment that "I honestly cannot believe that the Minister for Women would vote against women's safety."*[131]

> *"And that's what it all comes down to, safety. Because let's not kid ourselves—these campaigners do real harm to real people, all the time."*[132]

> *"They also protect women from conduct that has been recognised as violence against women."*[133]

128 Carey, A. (8 June 2018). NSW Minister for Women Tanya Davies Votes Against Abortion Clinic 'Safe Access Zones.' News.com.au. https://www.news.com.au/finance/work/leaders/nsw-minister-for-women-tanya-davies-votes-against-abortion-clinic-safe-access-zones/news-story/58e2e01454fa3b58d83c40c59a1960ed

129 Carey, NSW Minister for Women Tanya Davies Votes.

130 Carey, NSW Minister for Women Tanya Davies Votes.

131 Carey, NSW Minister for Women Tanya Davies Votes.

132 Carey, NSW Minister for Women Tanya Davies Votes.

133 Penovic, T. (15 Jun 2018). Explainer: What Are Abortion Clinic Safe-Access Zone and Where Do They Exist in Australia? *The Conversation.* https://theconversation.com/explainer-what-are-abortion-clinic-safe-access-zones-and-where-do-they-exist-in-australia-98175

> *"No person seeking lawful medical advice and care*
> *should be forced to run a gauntlet of abuse."[134]*

Verbal attacks against the MPs who chose to vote against the legislation could be labelled as the very harassment and threats that the majority profess to be trying to legislate against.

The same strategies used in surveying the community about decriminalisation are used in surveys about the issue of abortion clinic protesters. Questions are Alarmist and present a view of protesters as a danger to women and seek to elicit support for the safety of women. One survey undertaken in New South Wales demonstrated the success of getting people to "yes" with the framing of the question:

> *"Strong majority view (89%) that women seeking*
> *abortion should be protected from harassment or*
> *any form of threatening behaviour."[135]*

Safe access zone legislation does not only make reference to behaviours that the majority of the public would agree are inappropriate, such as harassing, threatening or intimidating, but also more benign behaviours including the following:

> *"Communicating by any means in relation to abortions in a manner that is able to be seen or heard by a person accessing, attempting to access, or leaving premises at which abortions are provided and is reasonably likely to cause distress or anxiety."[136]*

---

134 Penovic, Explainer.

135 Barratt, A., McGeechan, K., Black, K., Hamblin, and de Costa, C. (2018). Knowledge of Current Abortion Law and Views on Abortion Law Reform: A Community Survey of NSW Residents. *Australian and New Zealand Journal of Public Health.* 43(1):88-93. doi:10.1111/1753-6405.12825.

136 Parliament of New South Wales (2018*). Public Health Amendment (Safe Access to Reproductive Health Clinics) Bill 2018*, pg.2; Public Health and Wellbeing Amendment, Vic, 2015, pg.4.

In effect, this bans any and all communication of any kind related to abortion even if the person communicating such information is a relative or friend of the woman attending a clinic, and even if the nature of such communication is an attempt to provide support or information to the woman about her alternative options. This is very important when taken into consideration alongside the legislation of conscientious objection.

It is unclear how "reasonably likely to cause distress or anxiety" is interpreted or measured as there is no supporting evidence that women experience an increase in distress or anxiety when people are present outside a clinic.[137] It is however clear that whether the person actually experienced distress or anxiety is irrelevant as demonstrated by the case of a Victorian woman who was arrested, charged and convicted of an offence related to this law in 2016.

In a high profile case that went before the High Court of Australia, Kathy Clubb was charged with breaking the law in relation to the safe access zone by approaching a couple outside of an abortion clinic and providing them with a brochure. The charge against her was that she

> *"..did engage in prohibited behaviour, namely communicating about abortions with persons accessing premises at which abortions are provided, within a safe access zone, in a way that is reasonably likely to cause anxiety or distress."[138]*

The incident was video recorded and is described in the court documents:

---

137 Turner, J., Garratt, D. and McCaffrey, S. (1 Oct 2018). The High Court, Abortion Clinic Speech Restrictions and the Assessment of Harm. *The Western Australian Legal Theory Association.* https://walta.net.au/2018/10/01/the-high-court-abortion-clinic-speech-restrictions-and-the-assessment-of-harm/

138 Clubb v Edwards & Anor. Case M46/2018. High Court of Australia. https://www.hcourt.gov.au/cases/case_m46-2018

"The male of the couple is seen to speak and obviously decline the offering of the pamphlet and move, with the young woman, away. There is no evidence of duress or violence of any kind. The engagement between the Accused and the couple is brief and appears polite."[139]

The couple who were approached made no complaint and were not questioned by police, and no evidence was put forward that would suggest the couple were in any way intimidated or harassed by the defendant. Ms Clubb was convicted of the crime of communicating about abortion within a "safe access zone," in spite of the fact that no distress was caused and no complaints from the people involved were forthcoming. The court relied on the evidence of the video recorded incident, the testimony of the defendant who says, "*I believe I have the right to offer my help to women,*" and an abortion care psychologist who was not a witness to the incident.

Ms Clubb's conviction was subsequently appealed on the grounds of unconstitutionality of the law, in terms of its infringement on rights of free speech. This appeal failed and was elevated to the High Court. The legal arguments here revolve around whether the law banning communication about abortion within a "safe zone" constitute an unfair burden on political speech, and whether what Ms Clubb or others may do outside a clinic constitutes a political act. Whether such actions constitute an actual threat or causes any actual distress seems irrelevant to the appropriateness or fairness of the law. It would appear that the nature of this particular action of Ms Clubb's was indeed political as it was an orchestrated breach, wherein police were notified it would occur and they were present to both videotape the interaction and make the arrest.

139 Clubb v Edwards & Anor, High Court of Australia.

Evidence put forward to the High Court in the form of affidavits by two Experts, one a Director of one of Australia's largest abortion providers, and the second by a psychologist providing services at one Victorian abortion clinic, claimed that women are psychologically harmed by the presence of such activity. In their affidavits, they based their claims of harm to women on a number of studies undertaken in the United States.[140,141] The studies cited suffer from bias and serious methodological flaws.[142]

These claims have also been disputed in an article by myself and others in a published article which critically examined the evidence before the court.[143] We noted a number of deficiencies including the fact that none of the cited studies accounted for the variability of behaviour outside clinics, and that no significant differences in the emotional state of women presenting for abortion were able to be attributed to exposure to people outside. The questions asked of women were also biased in their language, asking about being *"confronted with anti-abortion protesters"* and *"to what extent did the protesters upset you, if at all?"* None of these studies could reliably conclude that 'protesters' harmed women, or had any lasting negative impact in relation to the abortion experience for women. One study, undertaken by Adherents, even concluded:

"Protesters do upset some women seeking abortion services. However, exposure to protesters does not

140 Foster, D., Kimport, K., Gould, H., Roberts, S., and Weitz, T. (2012). Effect of Abortion Protesters on Women's Emotional Response to Abortion. *Contraception,* 87:81-87.
141 Kimport, K., Cockrill, K., and Weitz, T. (2012). Analyzing the Impacts of Abortion Clinic Structures and Processes: A Qualitative Analysis of Women's Negative Experience of Abortion Clinics. *Contraception,* 85:204-210.
142 WECARE (n.d.). The Turnaway Study Analyzed by WECARE Director: The Latest Attempt to Reverse Evidence-Based, Women-Centered Advances in Abortion Policy. *World Expert Consortium for Abortion Research and Education* https://wecareexperts.org/content/turnaway-study-analyzed-wecare-director-latest-attempt-reverse-evidence-based-women-centered
143 Turner, Garratt, and McCaffrey, The High Court.

> *seem to have an effect on women's emotions about*
> *the abortion one week later.*"[144]

The transcript of court proceedings[145] demonstrates one way in which the veracity of Expert information is accepted as fact—"It is not necessary for the court to look at those studies"—while Discrediting the authors of a critique of the same studies; "I would personally, not call it an article."

> *"Now, your Honours, both Dr Allanson and Dr Goldstone referred to studies that they annexed to their affidavits that they said were supportive of the observations that they had made, personally, and the opinions that they had given formed on the basis of their qualifications. I am not going to take the Court to those studies. It is not necessary for the Court to look at those studies.*
>
> *Can I now, your Honours, respond to the appellant's attempt to rely on what has been described—although, I think, perhaps, inaccurately—as an article written by Dr Turner and two colleagues? It is a document published on a website. I would, personally, not call it an article. It does not appear to have been published in a journal, let alone a peer-reviewed journal."*

In the meantime, a woman who has been involved in the practical and emotional support of women with unintended pregnancies, and who states that by her presence outside the abortion clinic she is offering hope and another option, was fined $5000 and placed on a good behaviour bond.

---

144 Foster, Kimport, Gould, Roberts, and Weitz, Effect of Abortion Protesters.
145 Clubb v Edwards & Anor, High Court of Australia.

We cannot underestimate the distress that women may have been conditioned to experience when attending an abortion clinic by the way in which abortion workers framed the 'protesters'. Clinic escorts had become commonplace and women were advised that these were to protect them from people outside clinics, thereby perpetuating the idea that the activities of such people were threatening.

It is impossible to know how many women may have been assisted by the help offered by many outside abortion clinics or how many women now will not find out, until it's too late, what supports were available to them.

"I'm not sure how I would have managed without all the baby clothes, the cot, and even someone visiting me at home to make sure I was okay when I was on my own. It was amazing and I couldn't wait to volunteer in the pregnancy centre to be that someone for another woman." (Fiona)

Restricting Services

While White Ribbon may have been better advised to stick with their mission on violence rather than step into the abortion debate, it is not only such organisations that suffer for not toeing the line. For many women experiencing hardship during pregnancy and early parenting, pregnancy support agencies become a one-stop-shop for support, material resources, education, and sometimes even medical care. In Australia such agencies are few and far between, often managed by volunteers and relying on fundraising in local communities. This doesn't stop virulent attacks on them by Adherents who see the provision of support for any pregnant woman as a threat to abortion.

There are frequent attacks on such services both in the media and by politicians with many such organisations accused of lying to and manipulating women, although evidence of such claims is not usually forthcoming. In 2005, political attempts to force such groups to refer for abortion, or make it clear that they refuse to refer for abortion, failed.[146] The premise behind the Bill at the time was that pregnancy support services were being misleading and deceptive by not advertising services they do not provide,

---

146 Stott Despoja, N., et al. (2005). Minority Report: Transparent Advertising and Notification of Pregnancy Counselling Services Bill. https://www.aph.gov.au/Parliamentary_Business/Committees/Senate/Community_Affairs/Completed_inquiries/2004-07/pregnancy_counselling/report/d02

namely referral for abortion. More recently during the process of decriminalisation of abortion in Queensland, the State Health Minister claimed to be in receipt of recorded evidence that "major pro-life groups have been misleading women."[147] He stated that they were providing incorrect information to women and not declaring their position on abortion and that he had referred the matter as a formal complaint to the Ombudsman.

The only specific piece of information that made it to the media was that women are told they may have an increased risk of breast cancer by having an abortion, which he states "has been proven to be incorrect." While there is some evidence that abortion does not increase breast cancer rates, there is significant published research to the contrary, so "proof" of the former doesn't exist.[148] Whether in fact any person from any of the agencies actually told anyone this information cannot be confirmed at the time of writing. None of the agencies named have been in receipt of any specific information about what was recorded or when, so have had no opportunity to conduct their own investigation or defend their service.

All three of the services named by the Minister—Priceless House, Rachel's Vineyard, and Pregnancy Help Australia—have been active in Australia for more than a decade and provide a wide range of services to support women. Services include the provision of maternity clothing, baby furniture, parenting classes, post-abortive counselling programs and support groups, practical and emotional support. None of the three organisations claim decision making counselling as their primary work and all claim

147The Queensland Times (15 Oct 2018). Pro-Life Groups Caught Misleading Women, MP Says. *The Queensland Times.* https://www.qt.com.au/news/qld-health-minister-says-prolife-groups-are-mislea/3549713/
148 Deng, Y., Xu, H. and Zeng, X. (2018). Induced Abortion and Breast Cancer: An Updated Meta-Analyis. Medicine (Baltimore) 97(3): e9613. https://www.ncbi.nlm.nih.gov/pmc/articles/PMC5779758/

to provide only evidence-based information when they do.[149]

Yet based on assertions that "incorrect" information may have been provided on one or more occasions, the Health Minister has called for all three services to be shut down. This again places the focus of services primarily on the 'right' to abortion as opposed to a woman's right to access services she may need in order to continue a pregnancy.

One interview participant who volunteered her professional services at a pregnancy support centre stated:

> *"I hate being made to defend my work in supporting women because of someone else's ideological issue. How is giving a woman a pram and a shoulder to lean on an ideological service?"*

Another outside of Queensland stated:

> *"Our service has been targeted by a few individuals who question our ideological foundation, even when we are clearly providing practical and material support to families in the community. It is as though if we were found to be pro-life, we can't be trusted to provide a pram to a woman. This does have the potential to damage us in spite of the amazing reputation we have in the community."*

In 2013, with the help of a community working party of young mums, I established such a service in regional Victoria. The needs identified by the working party were specific and not related to abortion, but to the support needs of women and families in general in participating in the day-to-day life of the community with small children. These are the needs we set out to meet:

---

149 Personal communication.

- Provision of sheltered facilities at outdoor events where parents could safely sit in comfort to feed babies, allow toddlers to play, change nappies, or just rest from walking around.
- Infant massage and first aid for childrenclasses.
- Bringing baby home sessions where couples (or singles) learned valuable skills and knowledge to navigate those first few weeks at home with a newborn, including getting enough rest, juggling commitments, and staying connected in their relationships.
- Assisting dining facilities in the shopping district to become more family friendly by consulting on the provision of baby change facilities, feeding area for parents who need to sit and feed a baby, making room for prams, having toddler menus, and allowing families with toddlers to use toilet facilities.
- Other businesses, including real estate agents, banks, and retail shops, came on board the "family friendly community" program to provide seating for parents to feed babies, and toilets for toddlers to use.
- Regular get-togethers for dads to share and learn from each other during the pregnancy and parenting journey.
- Provision of prams, cots, car seats, and other essentials to assist families in need.
- Annual baby showers to collect all the essentials a new mum might need when she goes into hospital to have a baby. These were distributed by midwives, the maternity unit, local GPs and other community service organisations.
- Mental health assessments and referrals for women during the perinatal period.

These services were, over a period of years, brought under ideological attack by Adherents, including funding bodies, that expressed concern over the "right to life" agendas which had never existed. One would expect that every one of these services should be embraced by those who espouse "choice." Yet the service had funding withheld and was repeatedly undermined by people in the community who viewed the service suspiciously as "anti-choice." This was partly because of other aspects of my work which included educating the professional sector on assessing and managing mental health harms of abortion.

What this means is that the organisations struggled, and even years after I transitioned the organisation to its own community management, they continue the struggle of defending against ideological attacks that have no foundation in spite of their clear success in provision of services to thousands of families.

The deliberate strategy of Out-Grouping and Discrediting those who work in the provision of support and education to women experiencing challenging circumstances during pregnancy was made evident in an article in 2002 by one of Australia's longstanding Adherents, Leslie Cannold. She says:

> *"... this tactic can be undermined by the production of documentary evidence linking women-centred activists with the anti-choice movement and anti-choice beliefs. Presenting such hard evidence in the media enables questions to be asked about the motives women-centred activists have for denying their anti-choice connections and about their trustworthiness on other issues."*[150]

The "tactic" she refers to is what she calls the woman-centred strategy which she describes as being designed to undermine

150 Cannold, L. (2002) Understanding and Responding to Anti-Choice Women-Centred Strategies, *Reproductive Health Matters*, 10:19:171-179,

women's agency and depict women as irrational and fragile. Millar agrees with Cannold when she describes Dissidents who highlight concerns for women as "feigning concern" about women.[151] This is an interesting interpretation of the reality that most people working in such service provision simply note; that is that many women and families can do with some added resources and support when navigating pregnancy and parenting.

The strong message is that only Adherents can be trusted in their motives and in their actions to educate or support women, even though it is a very rare event that Adherents would be engaged in the establishment, funding, or support of services that provide genuine support. This perspective, of course, has been enshrined in laws that say only doctors with particular views can be trusted with women. It is enshrined in the academic sector when only researchers whose outcomes are consistent with Adherent views can be published. And it is enshrined in the media when only women who celebrate their abortions as a positive event can be heard.

The consequences of Alarmist Gatekeeping in restricting such services in the name of "rights" of course results in restricting rights that women may have to genuine choice. We know that most women seek abortion when they lack resources, yet the provision of resources is seen by Adherents as manipulative even when a woman hasn't expressed a desire for abortion.

The only possible conclusion one can draw is that Adherents appear to value only one decision, that is the decision to have an abortion. That decision must not be questioned, even to the extent of checking if there are other things that might meet her need so that she can make a different decision.

---

151 Millar, E. (2016). Mourned Choices and Grievable Lives: The Anti-Abortion Movement's Influence in Defining the Abortion Experience Since the 1960s. *Gender & History,* 28(2):501-519.

The New Backyard Abortion

Adherents claim that abortion rights are about the freedom of women to make choices to control their own reproductive function. Reproductive freedom in this sense, therefore, must include the right to contraception, abortion, pregnancy and parenting, and the right to change their mind about these options. Under this assumption the provision of a service that addresses the needs of women who change their minds after commencing a medical abortion should be embraced by Adherents. Of course, this isn't the case, given that such a phenomena would mean accepting that not all women are happy abortion decision makers, not all women feel fully informed, and not all women act from a position of freedom and autonomy in abortion decision making.

In 2013, Australia's inclusion of the drugs for medical abortion on the Pharmaceutical Benefits Scheme (PBS), making its procurement supposedly more affordable while being subsidised by tax dollars, was celebrated as a victory for women. It is worth noting that in spite of PBS listing of the drugs, abortion providers still charge hundreds of dollars for the provision of medical abortion, with many charging more for this than for the surgical option.[152]

---

152 At the time of writing Marie Stopes advertise the same price for both surgical and medical abortions, being "from" $440 each. https://www.mariestopes.org.au/abortion/

Abortion advocacy organisation Children by Choice acknowledge that "little is known about how much women's access to abortion has improved as a result of these changes" yet this doesn't stop Adherent efforts for greater expansion. Greater access arguments are often specific to women in rural and remote areas, which conflicts with the need for women to be able to access emergency medical care during a medical termination process.

Such efforts are replete with manipulative language designed to sell the process as an enhanced experience for women. Using soft language to describe medical abortion such as a "miscarriage," "natural," "in your control," or "menstrual regulation" are all designed to sell a product while manipulating the expectations of women who buy it. Among the selling points of medical abortion is that it supposedly puts the process back in the hands of women, under their control, and that it can be a more private process.

Yet many women have shared the horror of extreme pain, nausea, diarrhoea, and horrific bleeding along with recognising the unborn baby forced from their bodies among the frighteningly huge blood clots.

> *"They'd given me this sheet of things to look out for, bleeding through two pads etc.... but I didn't even read it properly... all I could think about was what I was doing and steeling myself to get through it. When the cramps started within 20 minutes of taking the second pills I thought, "this is manageable, I'll be okay." Within another 15 minutes I was doubled in agony with huge clots pouring out of me. I could feel them coming out.*

> *I'd rushed to the bathroom because I thought I was*

*going to be sick, then I sat on the toilet while all
this blood poured out. I didn't have my phone and
I couldn't get up to go and get it. I resigned myself
to the fact that I was probably going to die there, on
the toilet. I realised I probably deserved it when I
realised one of those 'clots' was my baby." (Chloe)*

One unique aspect of the process of medical abortion is that
women have an opportunity to consider what they have embarked
on with the time element between taking the two medications.
After ingesting the first drug, mifepristone, women wait 24-48
hours before taking the second drug, misoprostol, to complete
the abortion process. In the United States, amid urgent calls from
women who were expressing regret after taking mifepristone, a
small group of doctors began prescribing progesterone for these
women to counter mifepristone's effects. This service, Abortion
Pill Reversal, receives calls from hundreds of women every year
who are desperate to prevent their abortion. While not operated
within the rigour of a clinical trial, the service collected data on
more than 700 women which demonstrated a success rate up to
68% in pregnancy continuation, depending on the method of progesterone administration.

Calls for this service to be available to Australian women
began around the same time as the USA based organisation found
themselves fielding calls from many countries where they were
unable to provide the service. In 2015, after being contacted by
the US team, I established a small network of medical practitioners to provide progesterone for such women. With limited
human resources and no funding, the service was not actively
marketed or advertised in any way and relied on women who
may find the US service to be referred to me. While still in the
early stages of establishment I was contacted by a journalist from

Australian Doctor.

Australian Doctor is an internet and print magazine described as the "leading independent medical publication, informing, educating and engaging GPs for more than 30 years." It provides information on a wide variety of issues relevant to the health professions. The journalist wanted to ask me some questions about our service, which I politely declined as we were still navigating how best to provide service and didn't want promotion to mean a demand that we found difficult to meet. This didn't stop Australian Doctor from seeking Expert advice about the terrible dangers of what we were embarking on.[153]

Headlined with "Warning over medical abortion 'reversal' service," the service is introduced as being "offered by an anti-abortion group" and stated that it "has been condemned as dangerous and irresponsible."

The Expert quoted in the article is an experienced abortion provider and executive on one of the largest professional bodies in Australia for Obstetricians and Gynaecologists. It can therefore reasonably be expected that she has knowledge of the use of progesterone in early pregnancy, the fact that mifepristone does not cause a higher incidence of congenital abnormalities[154] and that women are often ambivalent about abortion and may change their minds or experience regret.[155]

---

153 Woodhead, M. (1 Dec 2015). Warning Over Medical Abortion 'Reversal' Service. *Australian Doctor.* https://www.ausdoc.com.au/news/warning-over-medical-abortion-reversal-service

154 Bernard, N., Elefant, N., Carlier, P., Tebacher, M., Barjhoux, C., Bos-Thompson, M., Amar, E., Descotes, J. and Vial, T. (2013). Continuation of Pregnancy After First-Trimester Exposure to Mifepristone: An Observational Prospective Study. *British Journal of Obstetrics and Gynaecology,* 120(5):568-575.

155 Garratt, D. and Turner, J. (2017). Progesterone for Preventing Pregnancy Termination After Initiation of Medical Abortion With Mifepristone. *The European Journal of Contraception and Reproductive Health Care,* 22(6):472-475.

Her comments in the article include aspects of both Alarmism and Disinformation.

> *"I would think that any Australian doctor who is prescribing a woman synthetic progesterone in this situation is acting very irresponsibly."*

> *"There was no way of knowing what effect progesterone would have in a woman who has recently taken mifepristone."*

> *"There is no evidence that this is an appropriate thing to do."*

> *"It would be highly dangerous to say that a pregnancy would proceed normally after that."*

> *"We don't have women suddenly changing their minds—this is basically not a problem; this is a furphy."*

These statements are also an attempt to Discredit those providing the service and, of course, denies the existence of women who change their minds. Which begs the question, what does it matter if the service exists if there are no women requesting it? Interestingly, there were a number of comments on the article from doctors who were critical of the Expert's assessment and Alarmism:

> *"Rather than being self-interested, this website appears to be offering women something for which there is no other option, without any self-reward or guarantee of success. Pity the rest of medicine (or perhaps just RANZCOG) doesn't want to get behind helping women at a time when they are so vulnerable."*

"I find it quite interesting that while pro-abortion supporters champion "women's choice," Royal Australian and New Zealand College of Obstetricians and Gynaecologists spokeswoman Professor De Costa's resistance to allowing doctors to offer the reversal treatment has the opposite effect of truly providing women free choice by discouraging their access to this form of treatment."

"highly dangerous"??? RANZCOG is on record for recommending (synthetic!) progesterone in early pregnancy for e.g. threatened miscarriage."

"Totally biased opinion given de Costa helped bring mifepristone to Australia... like asking a butcher if vegetarians get enough iron out of their diet.

Regardless of how much counselling a woman gets, she is permitted to change her mind. to say that she won't/can't is irresponsible and totally paternalistic."

Perhaps unsurprisingly, all the comments have since been deleted from the online version of the article.

In the United States, a number of state governments—Idaho, South Dakota, Arkansas, Utah, and Mississippi (at the time of writing)—have decided the risk versus benefit evidence of progesterone in this setting is convincing enough that they have legislated for women be told they have an option to reverse if <u>they change the</u>ir minds.[156] There is massive opposition to this

156 Bhatti, K., Nguyen, A. and Stuart, G. (2018). Medical Abortion Reversal: Science and Politics Meet. *American Journal of Obstetrics and Gynecology*, 218(3):315.1-315.6.

intervention from Adherents. The stated major objection is that there is not enough evidence to support the intervention.[157] It is likely, however, that underlying this objection is the concern that such interventions may threaten the Principle of abortion rights. Some of this opposition raises the issue of progesterone to counter mifepristone being a new therapy that does not yet have as strong an evidence base as many widely available medical interventions. However, all new and innovative medical interventions have a starting point, and this particular intervention is both low risk with potentially very high benefit.

While I am convinced that women should have access to such a remedy if they choose it, I am less confident that informing women about the possibility of reversal prior to commencing an abortion has any merit. In fact, such information may encourage anxious, ambivalent women to begin the process believing it can be stopped without fully understanding the risks they are taking.

In 2017, a case study article I had published on women who had accessed the service of Australian Mifepristone Reversal drew criticism from an Adherent who questioned the agenda of the service provision.[158] In a letter to the editor, the International Coordinator of a group called International Campaign for Women's Right to Safe Abortion called into question not only the peer review process for allowing the article to be published but also the agenda of the service providers.[159]

The author accuses the peer review process of enabling "anti-abortion efforts to dress up their political aims as science"

157 Grossman, D., White, K., Harris, L., Reeves, M., Blumenthal, P. D., Winikoff, B. and Grimes, D. A. (2015). Continuing Pregnancy after Mifepristone and "Reversal" of First-Trimester Medical Abortion: A Systematic Review. *Contraception, 92*(3):206-211
158 Garratt and Turner, Progesterone for Preventing Pregnancy Termination.
159 Berer, M. (2018). Response to "Progesterone for preventing pregnancy termination after initiation of medical abortion with mifepristone": what's the real point here? *The European Journal of Contraception and Reproductive Health Care*, 23(2):169-169.

and of "giving credibility of scientific publication when its underlying aim was to promote a way to stop abortion."

The service providers of Australian Mifepristone Reversal were accused of having the main purpose of finding "a clinical means to stop abortions already in process from taking place" with the suggestion that this is not the woman's expressed need. She further suggests that women who change their minds may have done so because they may have been exposed to health professionals who condemned them, showed them their ultrasound scan or "nasty visuals of chopped up foetuses." In Berer's mind there is no room for the fact that the women may simply have been extremely ambivalent or under pressure and subsequently sought, asked for, and consented to the service offered by Australian Mifepristone Reversal.

The journal's Editor responded strongly to this letter which was deemed to "level serious accusations at the editor and questions the reviewing process."[160] He went on to state that the published paper met all appropriate standards for research and publication and that rejection of it may have been considered to be censorship and suppression.

The Alarmist reaction by Adherents to this service is due to the perceived risk to the principle of abortion rights, yet underpinning that principle is meant to include the ideal that women have the right to full control of their own bodies. This must include the right to change their minds and access different treatments. Discrediting as "anti-choice" those services that provide women with added alternatives typifies the inconsistency and complete abstraction of the Dominant positioning.

Over almost five years of operation, the service has been contacted by close to 70 women who had taken mifepristone and

---

160 Bitzer, J. (2018). Answer to the letter of Marge Berer. *The European Journal of Contraception and Reproductive Health Care*, 23(2):170.

changed their minds. Almost all the women went to great lengths to contact the service, and then only after exhausting all other avenues of seeking help. One woman had visited three separate hospital emergency departments within the space of a few hours and been turned away, with one doctor telling her she should have thought about what she was doing before she did it. Many of these women were distressed and confused about why it was so difficult to find help and why the service isn't more widely promoted.

> *"I will always be pro-choice even though I wish I hadn't done this (started the medical abortion), but for women like me this should be part of our choice, surely?" (Becca)*

So far no typical scenario has been identified in women who change their minds and seek support, except for the common phenomena of immediate regret upon ingesting mifepristone. There have been women from every state of Australia who have accessed medical abortion via all means available, in private clinics, GP-prescribed, and by mail order. Every woman describes the moment that she realised she had done the "wrong" thing as a moment of complete clarity and often total panic.

About half of the women decide to proceed to termination after contacting the service. For those that talk about their reasons, they are usually succumbing to the same pressures that led them to abortion in the first place or their fears that mifepristone has damaged the unborn baby, something that is reinforced by abortion providers.

Around 80% of the women had first contacted or attempted to contact the abortion provider for advice. All but one of these was advised that they had no choice but to either continue the medical abortion process or attend the clinic to complete the abortion surgically. All were told that mifepristone would likely harm the unborn baby, which is not consistent with current evidence. Marie Stopes still has the following on the FAQ page on their website:[161]

> Q: What happens if I don't go through with the medical abortion?
>
> A: It is very important that you understand that mifepristone or misoprostol can damage a developing foetus. If you do not want to continue with the medical termination of pregnancy after starting, we strongly recommend that you have a surgical termination of pregnancy rather than continue the pregnancy.

This is not only untrue but provides added pressure for women to continue a process for which they have clearly withdrawn consent. For women whose pregnancies have continued, there is often an expressed disbelief that they could ever have considered aborting their now much-loved babies. For those whose pregnancies don't continue, the feedback has still been very positive with women expressing how thankful they were to have had an opportunity to "try to take it back."

---

161 Marie Stopes (n.d.). Medical Abortion. *Marie Stopes Australia*. https://www.marie-stopes.org.au/abortion/medical-abortion/

"To this day I regret going through with it and wish that I was five months pregnant. I think that I would love motherhood and I should never have let my family make such a big decision for me." (Aimee)

Silencing Creates a
Climate of Coercion

Alarmist Gatekeeping restricts information, leads to legislative change that disadvantages women needing support, and silences those who have negative experiences. All of these create an environment of coercion to one "choice" for women; abortion. Coercion can be a tricky phenomenon to measure and often presents as the existence of more than one factor that creates a sense of pressure. In the context of Alarmist Gatekeeping, the consequences of such manipulation of the Discourse mean we fail to see or speak out about the coercive nature of abortion even when it is most obvious.

Coercion is a contentious issue. Some argue that it exists so rarely that to discuss it is irrelevant. Others argue that abortion sought for social reasons is coercive in itself, whether or not the woman identifies it as such.[162] Attempts to highlight any negative factors for women around issues of abortion, whether they are potential adverse effects or coercive factors, are often dismissed as either completely false or anti-choice. Some Adherents go so far as to insist that when pro-life people talk about women who

162 Kramlich, M. (2003). The Abortion Debate Thirty Years Later: From Choice to Coercion. *Fordham Urban Law Journal*, 31:783; Grace, K. and Anderson, J. (2018). Reproductive Coercion: A Systematic Review. *Trauma, Violence, and Abuse*, 19(4):371-390.

regret abortion or change their minds about wanting abortions, such women are fabricated.[163]

This effort to relegate these stories to myth only serves to silence and stigmatise women who are suffering or who come to regret abortion. It also adds to the confusion or misinformed knowledge acquisition of those who may be called on to support clients who have experienced abortion negatively.

There is the occasional story of direct coercion that makes it into the media such as that of Jaya Taki who says her footballer boyfriend forced her to have an abortion, or the woman who told the Human Rights Commission her employer sacked her for not having an abortion.[164,165] The report on pregnancy discrimination released by the Australian Human Rights Commission in 2014 detailed many instances of pressure, coercion and lack of support for pregnant women.[166] With findings that around half of all women experienced discrimination during pregnancy or early parenting and that many experience what should be a joyous time as leaving them feeling "powerless, vulnerable and fearful" due to work insecurity, it is clear that such discrimination should be considered as an aspect of coercion.

Abortion providers themselves have admitted to knowing that women may be coerced. Carol Portman, a provider of late-term abortions in Queensland, attended Senate Hearings as part of her submission supporting decriminalisation of abortion in that state.

163 De Costa, C. (1 Dec 2015) *Australian Doctor Magazine*.
164 Sutton, C. (19 Mar 2017). Jaya Taki says NRL Star Tim Simona Partied After Her Abortion. *News.com.au* https://www.news.com.au/sport/nrl/jaya-taki-says-nrl-star-tim-simona-partied-after-her-abortion/news-story/
165 Bourke, E. (25 Jul 2014). Human Rights Commission Study Finds Widespread Discrimination Against Pregnant Women. *ABC News.* https://www.abc.net.au/news/2014-07-25/workplace-discrimination-against-pregnant-women-study/5623376?nw=0
166 Australian Human Rights Commission (2014). *Supporting Working Parents: Pregnancy and Return to Work National Review—Report.* https://humanrights.gov.au/our-work/sex-discrimination/publications/supporting-working-parents-pregnancy-and-return-work

She stated in part:

> *"Sometimes even in the best of circumstances we understand that a person is to a degree being coerced but feel they still need to go ahead, because it is their only choice, because otherwise this person will leave them, and their four kids (for example). It's very hard to know what to do in those circumstances so you go ahead with what their choice is even though to a degree they are being coerced."*[167]

Portman's statement to the committee raised no questions from the committee members and wasn't reported on in any mainstream media, leaving one wondering whether such practices are just so commonplace that we no longer notice them or we ignore them as they are too hard to face.

Let's consider other scenarios where women might attend for medical or surgical intervention and disclose that they are feeling pressured or coerced:

- Attending to undergo a breast enlargement saying her boyfriend has threatened to leave her if she doesn't go ahead. She doesn't really want the surgery but is scared so is 'choosing' it.
- A woman requests a tubal ligation saying her husband has demanded it even though she isn't really sure she wants to.

Would we be more outraged or ask more questions if doctors went ahead with such procedures, or would we simply accept that

---

167 Portman, C. (12 Sept 2018). In person submission to Queensland Senate hearings on Decriminalisation of Abortion. https://www.realchoices.org.au/2018/09/abortion-coercion-admitted/

in spite of such coercion it is ultimately considered the woman's choice and we should do what she requests even when stating she doesn't "want" it? With many stories around of women who have finished having children and who request a tubal ligation[168] only to be denied, we can be clear that the same criteria are not applied to any other medical or surgical procedure.

It isn't that Adherents don't acknowledge that reproductive coercion exists, more that they are preoccupied with what they consider to be "forced birth." The work they do on the coercion issue primarily concerns women who are victims of reproductive control such as contraceptive sabotage, sexual assault, and not being able to access abortion. Unsurprisingly Marie Stopes have a documented history of their preoccupation with women who can't get abortions while ignoring those who are forced to have them.

The latest offering from Marie Stopes was in 2018 when they released a draft White Paper entitled Hidden Forces: Shining a Light on Reproductive Coercion.[169] As expected from an organisation heavily invested in marketing and delivering abortion services, the paper has a strong emphasis on coercion related to continuation of pregnancies, with coercion to terminate barely warranting a mention. For the most part, coercion to terminate is no longer differentiated from coercion to continue a pregnancy, both being lumped together under the tidy label of "pregnancy outcome control."

The White Paper spends a lot of time within its fifty-plus pages lamenting the lack of a clear definition of coercion. I suspect this will remain a long-term problem for Adherents as they work to

---

168 Ford, C. (24 Jul 2016). It's 2016 and Women in Australia Still Aren't Allowed Control of Their Bodies. *Sydney Morning Herald.*
169 Marie Stopes Australia (2018). *Hidden Forces: Shining A Light on Reproductive Coercion: White Paper.* https://www.mariestopes.org.au/advocacy-policy/reproductive-coercion/

seek definitions that meet their ideological objectives of keeping abortion positively framed. Defining it will be hugely problematic when women often identify the very reasons they seek abortion as having been experienced as pressure or coercion.

While ignoring the prevalence of coercion toward termination, the White Paper makes a giant leap when it labels the Federal Government's 2006 pregnancy support counselling scheme a form of reproductive coercion because it doesn't allow abortion provider counsellors to access the Medicare rebate for counselling. They suggest that abortion providers, who only receive payment if a woman proceeds to abortion, demonstrate no bias in decision making counselling and should therefore have access to the payment.

There is a very interesting statement made in the midst of this section, in relation to pregnancy support counselling services: "In no other sector can such unregulated practices occur without legal ramifications." I would argue that in no other sector of health care can women receive a medical or surgical procedure for no reason other than that they request one, and doctors be forced to provide access to it either directly or indirectly.

Of course, the preference within this White Paper is that no doctor ever be allowed a conscientious objection to abortion because this too is considered a form of reproductive coercion. According to Adherents, women are autonomous, intelligent decision makers who don't need help or support in deciding whether abortion is right for them, but if they happen to come across a doctor who doesn't provide them with an immediate referral, they do not have the ability to simply locate a provider themselves and may be forced to "continue a pregnancy against her wishes or seek abortion at a higher gestation."

Little has changed in Marie Stopes' lack of attention to abortion coercion since their 2008 survey entitled Real Choices, seeking to understand women's experiences of unplanned pregnancy.[170] In their questions on why women resolved their unintended pregnancies in particular ways—parenting, adoption, abortion—their response options reveal exactly what they are looking for. Respondents were provided with multiple options as to how they might have been pressured into parenting or adoption but not a single option for an experience of pressure toward abortion. This alone typifies Adherents' lack of interest in abortion coercion and the reasons why it is vital that we now highlight the very real and very prevalent experiences of women pressured to terminate.

With leading abortion advocates and providers denying the existence of the dozens of women who change their minds every year after commencing medical abortions, we have a baseline for how Adherents view the existence or prevalence of coercion to terminate: these women simply don't exist.

> *"We don't have women suddenly changing their minds—this is basically not a problem, this is a furphy."*[171]

Most private abortion clinics operate on a walk-in, walk-out model. A woman phones to make an appointment and is scheduled for termination during the same appointment in which she may also receive information and/or counselling. Abortion advocates argue vehemently against alternatives such as ensuring at least two appointments with an opportunity between them to fully consider options, citing the added burden on women of two visits. Yet it seems possible there may be other benefits to abortion clinics in ensuring women only need to walk in the door

---

170 Marie Stopes International (2008). *Real Choices: Women, Contraception, and Unplanned Pregnancy.* https://www.mariestopes.org.au/wp-content/uploads/Real-Choices-Key-Findings.pdf

171 Woodhead, Warning Over Medical Abortion 'Reversal' Service.

once. The process was described by Felicity as a production line:

> *"The process was like being on a production line. Sit down, get a form, sit down, speak to a counsellor, sit down, have an ultrasound, sit down, move to another room, sit down... wait, wait, wait. Then finally it was done. And I felt nothing."*

There is a presumption by Experts that once a woman attends a clinic, she is there for an abortion regardless of her intent:

> *"By the time someone presents to an abortion service they have already weighed up all their options..."*[172]

Yet the experience of Meg tells a different story:

> *"Even though they said I could just start the abortion at the appointment, I went there with the intention of getting the information so I could go home and really think about it. I just didn't know what I wanted to do. Before I knew it, I'm sitting in front of this doctor with a pill in my hand and I'm still just thinking, hang on... then I put it in my mouth. When I walked out I think I was in shock. It wasn't until I was almost home that I suddenly became hysterical realising what I'd done. I had to pull over the car and I was vomiting on the side of the road and crying and crying."*

Arlo's story demonstrates how a woman can be pushed through the production line without a second glance, even after desperately seeking help from the abortion provider to help prevent her forced abortion. Arlo's boyfriend was outraged that she'd fallen pregnant, fearing that a baby at this stage of life would ruin his life, career, and future prospects. When persuasion wasn't

---

172 Rushton, This is what reproductive health experts think.

working, he resorted to threats of suicide.

> *"He booked the abortion. I rang them and told them what was happening, that I couldn't cancel, that I only wanted counselling when I got there. I told them that my boyfriend would come with me and he was forcing me. They promised to put a note on my file. When we arrived at the clinic I waited for someone to say something. The only time I was alone was when someone did the ultrasound but I didn't think that was the person I could talk to. All she said was "you'll be fine, this will be safer than childbirth." When I came out of that room and back to reception my boyfriend spotted me straight away and came to my side.*
>
> *They put papers in front of me to sign. I stared at the top saying "consent form." I felt desperate as he stood beside me waiting for me to sign. Desperate for someone to see my flagged file and take me aside, tell my boyfriend that I couldn't have the abortion for some reason. It never happened.*
>
> *I never had another moment without him by my side. When we sat with the doctor who barely looked at me but handed me that pills I felt like I was boring holes into her, willing her to see the note that I was promised would be there.*
>
> *My boyfriend drove me home and made me take the first pill before leaving me alone and going to work. I was defeated."*

As if it isn't horrific enough that a doctor would ignore a woman saying she felt coerced, women also describe direct coercion on the part of the doctor:

> *"I was crying, saying I didn't know what to do. The doctor just said, "Take the pill or get out," so I did. I don't even know why." (Hannah)*

> *"I had the pill in my mouth and I remember shaking my head and crying. I'm sure I was even saying I didn't want to, at least I was screaming it inside my head. The doctor just looked at me and said, "You can hardly bring such an obviously unwanted and unloved baby into the world, can you?" At that point of horror I swallowed. As soon as I got out of there I was already searching for a way to stop it." (Yvonne)*

These are not rare isolated incidents. Coercion is the norm that women live with, both from their circumstances, the people who are supposed to care about them, and the abortion providers who profess to uphold their rights.

> *"When I rang them after the abortion and I told them what they'd done, they said it was probably a good thing I'd had the abortion then, so I wouldn't still be with the guy." (Arlo)*

What is all the more horrific is that women like Arlo, Hannah and Yvonne are meant to be grateful for this "right" bestowed upon them, whether they want it or not.

"I did what everyone else thought was right for me but hind sight is always 20/20. I hope to be lucky enough to have another chance and to make it right."(Barb)

What Now?

"There is something wrong when something so big, so HUGE can happen before you even "get it." And I didn't "get it?" I thought there must be something wrong with me, but I guess not if it is happening to others.

Someone needs to sit you down, look you straight in the eye and be very clear about what you are doing, and make ABSOLUTELY sure you know what it means. Then you should be made to wait to make sure you REALLY know about it." (Tamra)

Yes, there is something wrong. Something so hugely wrong that it can be difficult to grasp it. Alarmist Gatekeeping provides a framework for seeing a huge manipulation at work. A manipulation which promotes an agenda through deception and which betrays women in the cruellest ways, when they are at their most vulnerable, and then expects them to be thankful.

As a society we are told that women will die without abortion, that women must have access to abortion if they are raped, that access to abortion is the only way in which women can experience equality with men, and that abortion is an expression of freedom and control of one's body.

The fact is that it is a fiction that any person has absolute autonomy and control of their own body. We have laws that govern many things we can and can't do and which impact us all day long. We must wear a seatbelt when travelling in a car, a helmet on a bike, clothing when we walk down the street. There are many times in life when we rely on others to support or resource us without this making us weak or unequal. Women's equality cannot be measured in its "sameness" to men. We are different, not lesser than. Women are not victims of biology, and to teach women such lessons is designed to make them feel inferior instead of feeling in awe of what their bodies can do.

Adherents frequently use the rarest situations of women who are raped and babies who will likely die during or soon after birth to promote an agenda of abortion at any stage for any woman for any reason.

They prioritise abortion rights above the actual experiences of women, using women's traumas to deny them their own reality in a way that sends a message that their children are disposable; that they are the price that needs to be paid in order for all other women to be equal.

They have managed to convince you to stay blind to the truth of it, to ignore your discomfort, and to continue the façade.

We live in a world where we attend baby showers, have gender reveal parties, call the unborn by names given to them while still in the womb when those babies are nurtured inside mothers who are well resourced and supported.

We turn a blind eye to those we are told are exercising "choice" when in fact they are frequently seeking any way out of a desperate situation and being forced onto a conveyor belt that ends only in abortion.

We don't want to hear the stories of these women because we might have to acknowledge our part in allowing a society that has ignored, reviled, and abandoned them.

We don't want to hear about foetal pain during abortion but we are pleased that our government sees fit to protect foetal animals from such cruelty. The National Health and Medical Research Council in the Australian Code for the Care and Use of Animals for Scientific Purposes states:[173]

> *3.3.10: Unless there is evidence to the contrary, it must be assumed that fetuses have comparable requirements for anaesthesia and analgesia as adult animals of the same species. Approaches to avoid or minimise pain and distress in the fetus must be designed accordingly.*

We grant human foetuses no such grace even knowing that the methods used in abortion are so barbaric that even politicians tasked with creating laws on abortion do not want to read about them.

We allow this 'equality' and 'rights' agenda to dominate our world view, dictate our legislation, remove rights from doctors and other professionals, and we wonder why so many women feel so alone and isolated.

---

173 National Health and Medical Research Council (2013). *Australian Code for the Care and Use of Animals for Scientific Purposes, 8th Edition.* Australian Government.

In my research and education work on the mental health impacts of abortion, I had always believed there could be common ground between abortion advocates and those who oppose abortion. While I had some awareness that there were tricky things to navigate in communicating about abortion and often addressed these in my writings, I really had no idea how pervasive and powerful the Dominant Messaging was until I undertook my PhD research.

I could (and still do) see different perspectives in the same stories and would wonder at how the Dominant presentation of a circumstance could be seen as supporting the need for abortion, while I saw it as supporting the need for better supports.

Two articles from the Dominant Discourse which speak to my own changing understanding of the Discourse demonstrate this. The first was from New Zealand about a young woman, Erica, who was denied an abortion at 18 weeks of pregnancy even though the law allows for abortion up to 20 weeks in certain circumstances.[174] The article was about promoting women's reproductive rights, through greater access to abortion and the need to change the law to allow unrestricted access.

The article quoted an abortion advocate who advises women what they should be saying in order to ensure their abortion request fits the criteria under New Zealand law. Erica describes experiencing suicidal thoughts after being denied an abortion, and says that she wasn't asked about her mental health history which should have allowed her an abortion. This is in spite of the evidence that having a history of mental health issues is a

---

174 Harris, S. (15 Oct 2017). Denied Abortion: Woman discovers pregnancy at 4 months, 2 weeks. *New Zealand Herald* https://www.nzherald.co.nz/nz/news/article. cfm?c_id=1&objectid=11928010

risk factor in increasing the risk of long-term psychological harm following abortion.[175] This latter point wasn't mentioned.

We also learn where Erica is now in her journey, although only as a passing curiosity as opposed to something of relevance. She has stopped drinking alcohol, given up smoking, is leading a healthier lifestyle, and while feeling "terrified," she also describes herself as "nervous" and "excited" to be welcoming her baby boy in a few weeks.

The second article presents the story of Sarah, whose baby received a prenatal diagnosis of Down Syndrome.[176] She did not consider termination and was clear about this to her medical practitioner at the start, asserting her own reproductive right to continue her pregnancy to birth. Sarah says she simply "got used to" medical professionals asking her to terminate her pregnancy as it happened so frequently. Another mother of a child with Down Syndrome says, "It was traumatic having to go in and say, "no, we don't want to kill our child" to every medical appointment."

While these stories seem to have little in common, the underlying theme and tension are substantially the same. Each deals with the issue of women's rights very differently, both abstracting the concept of rights from the actual experience of women, and both strongly advocating abortion. In Erica's case, even though she is now excited and looking forward to the birth of her son, a common change in perception when a woman does not procure

175 Coleman, P. K. (2011). Abortion and Mental Health: Quantitative Synthesis and Analysis of Research Published 1995-2009. *The British Journal of Psychiatry: The Journal of Mental Science*, 199(3):180–186. https://doi.org/10.1192/bjp.bp.110.077230; Fergusson, Horwood, and Ridder, Abortion in young women and subsequent mental health.
176 Brook, B. (9 Oct 2017). They called me an idiot and said I should abort: The anguish of a prenatal diagnosis. *News.com.au.* https://www.news.com.au/lifestyle/health/they-called-me-an-idiot-and-said-i-should-abort-the-anguish-of-a-prenatal-diagnosis/news-story

an abortion, the 'problem' that she couldn't or didn't abort is the focus.

Sarah and the many parents who welcome, love, and value their children with Down Syndrome have to fight for their right to birth their babies. Their fight doesn't end there. There is pressure to end the lives of the 'less than perfect' through earlier access to prenatal testing, and pressure to terminate when there is an adverse diagnosis. This broad, ongoing social hostility means they are fighting for the very existence of their children even after they are born. Many lament the messages their children receive about the value of their lives as they become aware of the messages that they should never have been born.[177]

Even when faced with such stories the majority of the public (Incognisants) will believe the Dominant Messaging. The real stories of women are much more complex and nuanced and are rarely about life-saving needs, but about inequities in life that don't accommodate the facts of their biology.

Naming Alarmist Gatekeeping, identifying the individual strategies, and developing critical thinking about all the ways in which it manifests is only a very small step and will be meaningless if we continue to self-censor or allow ourselves to be silenced.

The more people who begin to ask questions, who are prepared to move through the discomfort of what they have previously ignored or not known, the more difficult it is for those in control to maintain the censorship.

When you consider the story of the "wrong twin terminated" and feel horror or sadness or dismay, ask yourself why this baby,

---

177 Personal communication, Mother of child with Down Syndrome, June 2018.

this loss, is different from the hundreds of late-term abortions done every year on healthy babies.

> *"If it hadn't been legal then maybe I would be awaiting the arrival of my child instead of being down and depressed and guilty every day. I needed help. I didn't need an abortion. I see that now." (Amanda)*

When you read an article about women having abortions to escape domestic violence or because they are struggling financially, ask yourself whether situations like these seem to be acts of freedom, autonomy, equality. Or whether abortion becomes an act of desperation because few people are offering a genuine alternative.

If you have read all of this book and at least considered the information and believed the women, you can no longer at any time say that you didn't know. It is important not to shy away from the discomfort of learning new information or old information in a new way. No matter the path you have taken or decisions you've made based on prior information, everything you do from this moment forward can be different and can contribute to a more positive and supportive culture.

Afterword

Dismantling Alarmist Gatekeeping Strongholds

Since unveiling Alarmist Gatekeeping as a theory, I've been surprised at how many researchers have come forward excitedly talking about how this theory fits their field of research. It should disturb us all that such manipulative and powerful strategies are being utilised to control our thoughts and our actions in so many different areas. Even more disturbing is the way in which legislative changes are being made so quickly, on so many issues, with little evidence, but a whole lot of rhetoric.

When Alarmist Gatekeeping Discourses are at play, it is clear there are hidden harms about which many people remain silent, but that are significant and life changing. How do we know if what I think I know about an issue is true, or whether I have been manipulated by Alarmist Gatekeeping? Firstly, look at the Dominant Messaging:

- On what evidence is the position based?
- What is the alternative evidence?

- Who provides the alternative evidence and what happens when they do?
- Am I required to change my language in order to accommodate the Dominant view?
- What happens when I refuse?
- Does it feel risky to talk in opposition to the Dominant Discourse?
- Am I made to feel I am in the Out-Group when I don't wholeheartedly embrace the allowed view on an issue?
- Are organisations which appear to have no vested interest in a specific controversial issue putting out statements or developing policy that supports the Dominant Messaging and leaves no room for debate?

On the issue of euthanasia, Adherents tell us that we must have laws to allow assisted dying because otherwise "people have little option but to die slowly and agonisingly." Marshall Perron's desire was to change the law to allow euthanasia using emotive Alarmism, "to bring to an end the torture many endure on the death bed."[178]

We see here the Recruiting language. How could anyone want someone to die so tortured? Why wouldn't you vote "yes" to such a law so that people had a different option? Yet, is this the reality? When the Victorian government legislated in favour of assisted dying, it was estimated that around a dozen people would utilise the service in the first year.

In reality, more than 120 people ended their lives under this new legislation. Their reasons were rarely about dying torturously or in agony, but about loss of autonomy, being unable to engage in activities of enjoyment, and loss of dignity.[179] How

178 Perron, M. (1995). *Hansard*: Extract from the Parliamentary Record 22 February 1995. Rights of the Terminally Ill Bill. https://parliament.nt.gov.au/__data/assets/pdf_file/0003/367950/extracts.pdf
179 Woodley, M. (2 Sep 2020). Voluntary Assisted Dying Report Released. *NewsGP.* https://

many would have voted to allow assisted dying in these cases? Perhaps a few, but certainly less than were caught up in the Alarmism of fictitious torture and agony.

Other researchers are applying my theory of Alarmist Gatekeeping to areas of gendered narratives of domestic violence, gender ideology, climate change, poverty among university students in Canada, home-schooling in Wales, and many more. Many of these issues have at their core individual rights and freedoms that can be impinged on, perhaps unintentionally, while the principle at issue becomes held as more sacred than the people who may be impacted. The greater lesson here for all of us is to always critically question that which is put before us. We must always make sure we examine all of the evidence while watching closely for how people are treated when they try to engage in debate.

For women today, it is incumbent on all of us to do what we can to ensure our communities are places where women can feel encouraged and supported enough to withstand the very real pressures telling them that without abortion, their equality is not guaranteed and their worth is less. We ensure equality by valuing and accommodating our differences, not by forcing any group to endure consequences of impossible decisions.

We begin by recognising and calling out Alarmist Gatekeeping when we see it. We offer alternatives and develop GateBreakers; that is, statements of truth and evidence on an issue that provide the alternative information.

As more researchers identify the Alarmism and Disinformation inherent in their fields, GateBreakers—designed to name and expose the strategies and present the factual alternatives—can be developed and widely disseminated.

Look out for my next book,

'Gatebreaking: Countering Alarmist Gatekeeping'

which outlines concrete strategies to respond to and counter the disinformation and manipulation inherent in such controlled discourse. Above all, we must gain strength in numbers by refusing to self-censor and encouraging debate even when it makes us uncomfortable.

Keep up to date with my other writings at:

www.debbiegarratt.com

Glossary

Abortion: A procedure undertaken on a pregnant woman that has the direct intention of ending the life of the foetus.

Abstraction: A strategy used to draw attention away from information that may threaten the Underlying Principle. Abstraction seeks to prioritise and generalise the Underlying Principle as an end in itself and Decontextualise the Principle from the reality of its enactment or outcome.

Adherents: People who are in conscious agreement with and uphold the Dominant Discourse Principle. Only Adherents have the power to decide who is in their group.

Agnotology: A term coined by Robert Proctor to describe the study of ignorance.

Alarmist Recruitment: The discourse atmosphere created by the use of Obfuscation and Abstraction. It is also a strategy through which the perception of the public is controlled to ensure that the Underlying Principle is upheld.

Censoring: Process of exclusion of information that is perceived to threaten the Underlying Principle using strategies of Silencing from the public discourse, and defining acceptable language.

Discrediting: Together with Out-grouping, Discrediting is used to undermine those in the out-group either professionally or personally in order to create doubt and disbelief in their attempts to contribute to the discourse. Negative attributes of character and motive are ascribed to those in the out-group.

Disinformation/misinformation: In this study, Disinformation is used to describe intentionally untruthful or incorrect information. Misinformation is Disinformation that is diseminated by those who may not know it to be factually incorrect. It is not always possible to know whether the proponent of information knows for sure the factual basis of what they are saying, however assumptions are made in the study that when a person 'should' know by virtue of their position or education that what they say is Disinformation when factually incorrect.

Dissidents: People who either disagree with the Dominant Discourse or who have been Out-Grouped as such by Adherents.

Dominant Discoursing: This encompasses the dominant public communications on a specific issue which is in some way polarising and which exercises control "by one group or organisation over the actions and/or the minds of another group, thus limiting the freedom of action of the others, or influencing their knowledge, attitudes or ideologies".[180]

---

180 Van Dijk, T. (2013). Discourse, Power and Access. In Caldas-Coulthard, C. R. and Coulthard, M. (eds.), *Texts and Practices: Readings in Critical Discourse Analysis,* Taylor and Francis, pp 93-113.

Experting: The process of promoting an Influential Person as an expert on the Underlying Principle whether or not they have particular 'expertise,' but by virtue of their agreement with the Principle. An organisation may be Experted by publishing a policy statement that upholds the Principle, even if that organisation has no direct connection to the Principle issue.

Illusory-Truth effect: Named and observed by researchers in the 1970s, this describes the tendency for people to believe as true information that is often repeated and which therefore becomes familiar.

Incognisants: People who uphold the Dominant Discourse Principle whether or not they specifically agree with the entirety of the perspective, because they have passively internalised the Dominant Messaging as true.

Influential People/Person: An Influential Person is always an Adherent and has some prominence in the field of promoting the Principle. They may be a leader of an Adherent organisation or some other person with a public profile who has always promoted the Dominant Discourse position. They are experted on the issue even if they have no specific expertise other than that they strictly adhere to the Underlying Principle.

Managing Perception/Balancing Risk: Perception and risk are interrelated for practitioners, with balancing risk involving the management of perception. Perception includes the way in which clients, colleagues or any other person may interpret information provided by the practitioner.

The risk is assessed based on perception factors, personal values, and professional responsibilities.

Obfuscating: Refers to statements used in strategic ways to persuade people to agree with the Underlying Principle. This is a quality of the Discourse that is comprised of the dissemination of Disinformation (information that isn't true), Misinformation (unwitting dissemination of Disinformation), and Inconsistency (the prevalence of inconsistent and often confusing information).

Out-Grouping: The categorisation of people in disagreement with the Dominant Discourse, or people who use Taboo Talk that is perceived to threaten the Underlying Principle of the Discourse, as both a minority and a negative force.

Panopticism: Process of internalised self-monitoring (censoring) based on the belief or concern that one is under constant scrutiny.[181]

Perspective Gatekeeping: Conceptualises the action and power of Adherents to control the perspective, views, beliefs and behaviours related to upholding the Underlying Principle. It involves processes of Viewpoint Discrimination and Censoring.

Pervasive: Meaning that the Dominant perspective is apparent across a wide range of influencing spheres including, but not limited to media, education institutions, professional bodies and legislation.

181 Foucault, M. (1991). The Order of Discourse. In M. Shapiro (Ed). *Language and Politics*. Oxford: Basil Blackwell Publisher Ltd, pp 108-138.

Strategic Ambiguity (also see Unified diversity): A process of using ambiguous statements that encourage agreement on a vague and abstract message. Such agreement may then be misrepresented as agreement on more specific issues. For example: "We all want women to have equal opportunities" can be reframed to suggest agreement that women need access to abortion for this to occur.

Toeing the Line: To Toe the Line means to comply with the expectation of the Dominant Discourse to uphold the Principle, doing and saying nothing that is a real or perceived threat to the Principle. Whether a person toes the line effectively is determined only by Adherents. Practitioners may Toe the Line by Self-censoring, that is by withholding, or modifying information or by Opting out, by not engaging at all with women who disclose abortion.

Underlying Principle or Principle: This refers to the particular perspective or ideal that dominates the way in which the issue is discussed.

Unified Diversity: Related to Strategic Ambiguity. A way of describing a general abstract agreement among many within which there may be diverse agreement or disagreement on the detail or specifics.

Viewpoint Discriminating: The preferment and promotion of the voices of Influential People described as experts by Adherents within the discourse. This includes a process of Out-Grouping and Discrediting those who disagree with the Dominant perspective.

www.ingramcontent.com/pod-product-compliance
Lightning Source LLC
Chambersburg PA
CBHW060334030426
42336CB00011B/1337